Back in Line

To Peter and Elizabeth

Back in Line

Jean Oliver MSCP, SRP

Chartered Physiotherapist, Back Clinic, Cambridge, UK

Drawings by Ann Blythe

Anatomical illustrations by Jean Oliver

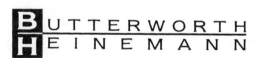

OXFORD   AUCKLAND   BOSTON   JOHANNESBURG   MELBOURNE   NEW DELHI

Butterworth-Heinemann
Linacre House, Jordan Hill, Oxford OX2 8DP
225 Wildwood Avenue, Woburn, MA 01801-2041
A division of Reed Educational and Professional Publishing Ltd

  A member of the Reed Elsevier plc group

First published 1999

British Library Cataloguing in Publication Data
A catalogue record for this book is available from the British Library

Library of Congress Cataloguing in Publication Data
A catalogue record for this book is available from the Library of Congress

ISBN 0 7506 2872 3

Endorsed by the OCPPP
Printed and bound in Great Britain by Martins the Printers,
Berwick on Tweed

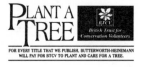

Contents

Preface

With so many books about backs on the market, you would think that by now we would have got to grips with the problem. But in fact the opposite is true: back pain is on the increase. Despite the fact that a lot of brilliant research has been done on the subject, the findings have not reached the people who need it most – those who have the back pain!

The purpose of this book is to give you the benefit of this research, which will throw new light on the cause of *your* back pain, so that you are able to understand your particular problem and will then know how to deal with it.

You may have found already that your back or neck problem differs in some ways from other people's, that what has helped someone else's back has not necessarily helped yours, and wondered why this was so. *There is more than one solution to back and neck problems because there is more than one cause*, and this is the main message of this book. Because the spine differs in shape from person to person and the amount of suppleness each of us possesses varies, it is not surprising that one person's spine will react in a different way from another person's spine to the stresses and strains of everyday life. These differences help to explain why some people, for example, will prefer to stand or walk in order to relieve their back pain, while others will prefer to sit down.

In the past, most self-help guides to dealing with back pain have taken the view that general advice and indiscriminate exercises should solve everyone's problem and, if they don't, then it is the patient's fault for not following the advice or for not doing enough exercise. This 'hit and miss' approach has failed because what most people with back pain need is *specific* advice for their particular problem.

All too often, back pain returns, seemingly for no reason – at least, for no apparent reason. Although therapy may sometimes help you to overcome a bout of back or neck pain, there is no evidence that it can prevent it recurring. However, my many years of treating patients suffering from back and neck problems have shown me that, given a clear understanding of what has gone wrong with their back and with specific advice, most people *can* relieve their pain and are often able to prevent their problem returning.

Why the title, *Back In Line?* This has been chosen because so many of our spines are out of line; in other words, the angulation (or alignment) between the bones is poor. It used to be thought that small defects, such as one leg being slightly longer than the other, one hip slightly higher than the other or one foot turned out more than the other, were unimportant. We now know that this is not so, and that even small defects in the angulation of the feet and legs can alter the alignment of the spine, causing repetitive stresses on it which add up over the years. Because they are small, these defects are often overlooked as an important cause of back pain.

We all possess a body with its own particular shape, often resembling that of one of our parents or grandparents. People frequently make comments like, 'He stands just like his father' because we have inherited a bone structure which makes us more inclined to stand in one way or another. Defects that may be small in our youth usually become more accentuated in adulthood, so that over the years we literally change our shape. You only have to look at an old photograph of yourself to see this. The change has occurred because of the way we have used our bodies. The way we have habitually sat, stood, walked, lifted etc. influences our body shape, perhaps resulting in our becoming a bit stooped, standing crookedly and then walking unevenly, without realizing it. The change happens so slowly that we hardly notice our alignment altering. But this change – slight though it may be at first – alters the way that we move, sometimes making our spines more vulnerable to even minor stresses. If one of the tyres on a car is flatter than the others, the car will be lopsided and will move differently, wearing out more quickly than it would have done otherwise. And so it is with our bodies: they work far more efficiently if they are used in a balanced way. Perhaps the day will come when this important information is taught in schools, before bad habits are formed. This book has been written so that you can discover how you can help your own back problem by getting it *Back In Line*.

Jean Oliver

Acknowledgements

I would like to acknowledge the invaluable part played by the late Jacquie Scott of the Haslemere Sports and Physiotherapy Clinic, in convincing me of the relevance of alignment in the treatment of back problems. Jacquie's thinking was way ahead of others in this respect and it was through her that I met Paul Barcroft, the Managing Director of The Langer Biomechanics Group (UK) Ltd. Paul's tuition in biomechanics, and his support during my experiments with the use of orthotics, increased my understanding of this exciting field and have been of inestimable benefit to me and my patients. I am also grateful to Joanne Farmer, also of Langers, who had the important task of evaluating my biomechanical measurements.

I would also like to express my gratitude to Ann Blythe for her enlivening drawings, and for her patience and interest in the whole concept of this book.

Many of the tips included in this book are from patients I have treated over the years, and from my ever-resourceful physiotherapy colleagues, Alison Middleditch in particular.

I would like to pay tribute to David Hewerdine for his help in overcoming my fear of computers and also for passing on to me his enthusiasm for their beneficial use, and to the late Margaret Hewerdine for reading through the text and making useful corrections.

Finally, my thanks go to my husband, Peter, and daughter, Elizabeth, for their tolerance during my long sessions in the computer room.

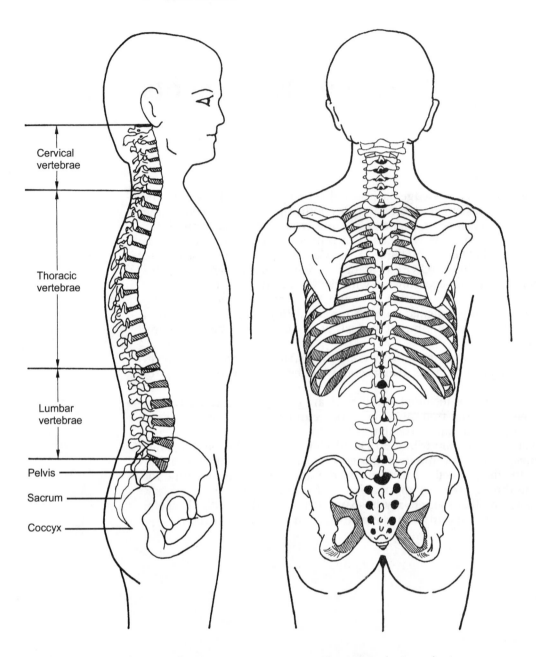

Cervical
vertebrae

Thoracic
vertebrae

Lumbar
vertebrae

Pelvis

Sacrum

Coccyx

Fig. 1.1 Side view of spine.   **Fig. 1.2** Back view of spine.

1
How the back works

Most back and neck pain originates in the spine itself, even though you may not necessarily feel it down the centre of your spine. Therefore, if you understand how the spine works, it will help you to deal with your problem.

Structure of the backbone (spine)

At first sight, the spine looks complicated (Figs 1.1, 1.2) but in fact it consists of a series of bones called **vertebrae** (Figs 1.3, 1.4) joined together by discs.

The front of the spine

The front parts of the vertebrae resemble a child's building blocks, stacked one on top of the other. The discs act as shock absorbers, cushioning the spine from jolts from the legs as we walk, step off kerbs, run, jump, and so on. The discs have an outer fibrous casing called the **annulus**, while the inside is a gel called the **nucleus**. When weight is taken through the spine, the nucleus spreads out and the annulus bulges slightly like a car tyre (Figs 1.5, 1.6).

The discs allow movement to occur between the vertebrae. When we bend forwards, the back of the disc (which also happens to be its weakest part) is stretched and becomes thinner, causing the nucleus to be positioned further backwards in the disc (Fig. 1.7). When we lean backwards the nucleus may be positioned slightly forwards (Fig. 1.8).

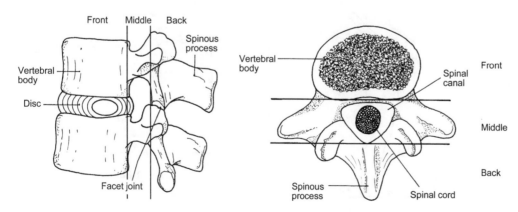

Fig. 1.3 Side view of part of spine.

Fig. 1.4 Cross-section through spine.

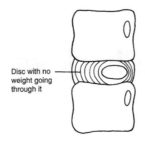

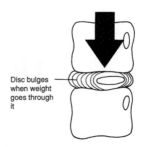

Fig. 1.5 Unloaded disc: side view of spine.

Fig. 1.6 Loaded disc: side view of spine.

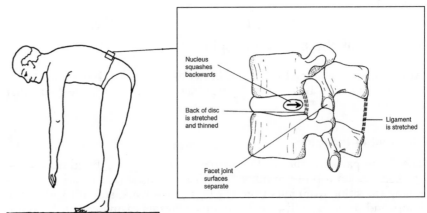

Fig. 1.7a Forward bending.

Fig. 1.7b

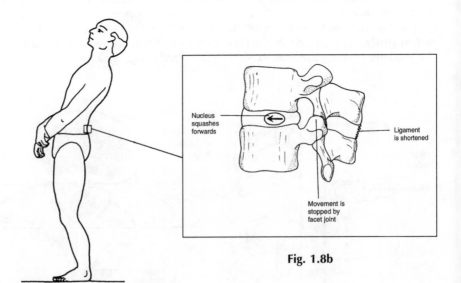

Fig. 1.8b

Fig. 1.8a Backward bending.

The height of the discs changes throughout the day. This is because there is a lot of fluid inside them, some of which is squeezed out when pressure is put through them (Fig. 1.9). This happens particularly when we lift or sit in a slouched position. Consequently, by the end of the day, our spines are usually about a centimetre shorter than when we wake up in the morning. When there is less pressure on the discs, for instance when we lie down, water is gradually sucked back into them and they swell up again.

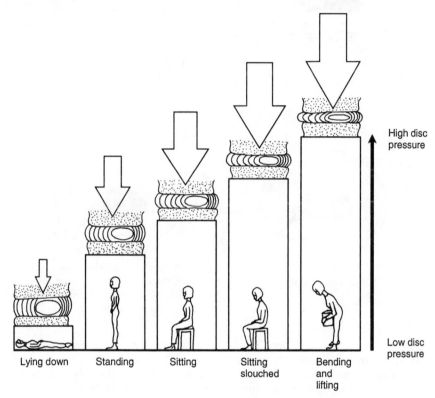

Fig. 1.9 How pressure on the discs is affected by different postures. (Adapted from A. Nachemson, 1976. The lumbar spine: an orthopaedic challenge. *Spine*, **1**, 59–71.)

Varying the amount of pressure that goes through our spine during the day is important, and keeps our discs healthy. When fluid is sucked into our discs, it brings with it food substances and oxygen; when fluid is squeezed out of our discs it gets rid of waste products. So it is not good for our backs if we sit all day: it is much healthier to give our backs some variety, to sit for a while, then walk a little.

Injuries to the discs are fairly common (*see* pp. 17–28). Strains caused by repetitive bending, twisting and lifting (Fig. 1.10) add up over the years and may cause disruption and tears in the back of the disc, its weakest part.

The back of the spine

The back part of the spine controls movements. On both sides of the discs are small joints called **facet joints** which fit together snugly to prevent you from overstretching your discs by leaning back too far or twisting

Stages of disc damage

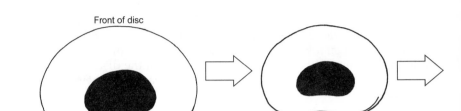

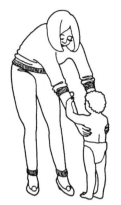

Fig. 1.10 Repetitive bending, twisting and lifting – the most dangerous combination of movements for the discs.

Fig. 1.11 A healthy disc (cross-section).   **Fig. 1.12** Disruption of fibres at the back of the disc.

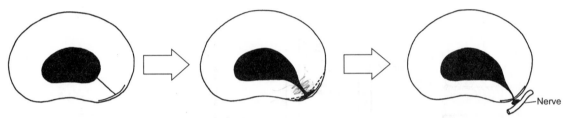

Fig. 1.13 Tears in annular part of the disc.

Fig. 1.14 A bulging disc: nucleus travels down one of the tears.

Fig. 1.15 A prolapsed disc: the nucleus has burst through the outer annulus and is pressing on a nerve causing 'sciatica' (pain in the leg).

excessively. However, when we bend forwards, the facet joints unlock and allow more twisting to occur (*see* Fig. 1.7). This is why, if we twist at the same time as we bend, the discs become more vulnerable. As with all joints, the facet joints can suffer from 'wear and tear' (*see* p. 29).

Ligaments are cords or sheets of fibrous tissue which join the bones together, giving stability to the spine. By being highly sensitive to being stretched, the ligaments also have a protective function: if we overstretch them they become painful. Some people's ligaments are longer than average, allowing greater movement in their joints; these particular ligaments may also be weaker and therefore more easily injured (*see* p. 12).

Projections of bone such as the **spinous processes** provide attachments for these ligaments and muscles. You can actually feel the ends of these processes just under your skin in the midline of your back, so you can imagine how deep all the other structures are.

The middle of the spine

The middle of the spine consists of a long, bony/ligamentous tube called the **spinal canal** (Fig. 1.4). Through this runs the **spinal cord**, an important structure which is a collection of nerves originating in the brain. Two nerves are given off from the spinal cord at the level of each disc, one nerve going to the right side of the body and the other to the left. Each nerve goes to a specific area of the body. The nerves have a number of functions – including making the muscles work and transmitting the sensations of touch, heat, cold and pain back to the brain so that we can experience them.

The muscles

The spine is completely surrounded by **muscles** – not just behind but also at the side and in front (the abdominal or 'tummy' muscles). When muscles are relaxed they are soft. The purpose of the muscles is two-fold: (1) to keep your spine stable so that your arms and legs can move efficiently; and (2) to move your spine. In order to do this they contract, or shorten, and become firmer. This also has the effect of putting pressure through your spine. Instructions to make the muscles contract travel from your brain through the nervous system. The more the muscles contract, the more pressure is put on your spine. While a certain amount of pressure is good for your spine, too much pressure can be harmful.

Two things can bring about this harmful increase in pressure: (1) excessive *physical* pressure caused, for example, by sitting for prolonged periods or lifting weights that are beyond your back's capacity to cope with; and (2) excessive *psychological* pressure. This does not mean that the pain is 'all in the mind'; far from it. In fact, it is impossible to imagine that you have pain. But anxiety makes your muscles tense up, often without you realizing it, and the rise in muscular tension increases the pressure on your discs.

Back pain causes some muscles to weaken – especially the abdominal (tummy) muscles – and other muscles to become hyperactive or to go into spasm and tighten. They then feel hard to the touch. This creates an imbalance which causes abnormal stresses on the spine (Fig. 1.16). This is why exercises to restore muscle *balance* play an important part in preventing back pain or in recovering from it. It is all too easy to work hard at strengthening the wrong muscles!

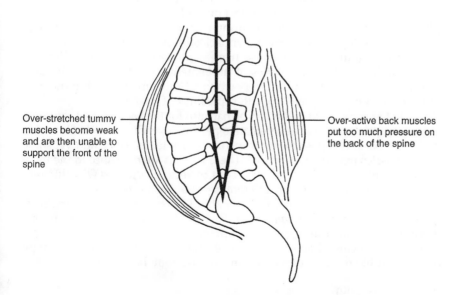

Over-stretched tummy muscles become weak and are then unable to support the front of the spine

Over-active back muscles put too much pressure on the back of the spine

Fig. 1.16 The effect of muscle imbalance on the spine.

Movements of the spine

The basic movements of your spine are bending forwards and backwards, sideways bending, and turning to the right and left, but there are many combinations of these basic movements. They occur all through your spine, but certain areas of your spine are naturally more supple in some directions than in others. For example, near the top of your neck there is a lot of turning movement, while in the middle of your neck and at the base of your spine there is more flexibility in forward (especially) and backward bending. These are the areas that are more likely to suffer from wear and tear.

Two other very important movements occur in the spine which affect its length: compression and distraction. The spine is compressed, in particular, when we sit, lift or carry objects, and also if we are over-anxious (*see* p. 5). On the other hand, when we stand or – especially – lie down, the spine regains some or all of its normal length.

The fact that the spine is able to move so freely allows the arms to stretch more and increases the stride length of your legs. When you have back pain you notice immediately how tiny movements of your arms or legs can set off the pain.

As we all know, babies are very supple. As we get older, we tend to stiffen up a little. Some people are naturally more supple than average (*see* p. 12); others are born with shorter ligaments which makes their joints naturally stiffer. No matter how much stretching the stiffer people do they never become excessively supple, that is, without damaging themselves in the process. It is useful for everybody to know what their particular body type is so that they do not force movements that are unnatural for their body.

Exercises

Every day we perform thousands of movements with our arms, legs and head. Most of these movements affect our spines in some way. For example, simply moving one leg in front of the other, as when walking, involves moving many joints and muscles in our spine.

What distinguishes an exercise from a movement is simply that, by definition, an exercise is a series of movements 'performed for the sake of health'. Were we to do the proper type of movements during the day, our backs would get plenty of the right kind of exercise.

But just as some movements can be harmful for the back, so also can some exercises, and these vary from person to person depending on what is wrong with their back. It is possible for someone's back to *feel* weak, and yet some of the muscles may be hyperactive. There is often an imbalance in the muscles that control the spine, and this needs correcting, which is why different exercises need to be done for different types of back problems.

Exercises should *not* be painful, nor should they cause pain afterwards. *If any exercise you do does cause pain, then STOP doing it at once.* Pain is a warning that you could be doing damage.

In the following chapter, different exercises are shown for each type of back problem. The purpose of an exercise may be:

- to relieve pain;
- to strengthen muscles;

- to stretch tight structures;
- to help correct your posture.

How often should exercises be practised? It depends why the exercises are being done. If the exercise is to *relieve pain*, do it as often as you can, every hour if necessary. As a general rule (unless otherwise stated), *stretching* exercises should be done four times, twice a day, and *strengthening* exercises should be done twice or three times a day, ten times each. The exercises will help to restore good posture and movements, and should be carried out until you are moving your back properly. However, it is important that you only do exercises that are right for *your* back. The wrong exercises can do more harm than good. Our backs change as we get older, and periodically you may find it helpful for a chartered physiotherapist to check that you are still doing the right kind of exercises to suit your back.

Muscles work better if they are warmed up before being exercised. Especially first thing in the morning if your back is very stiff, warm up your back by standing with your back under a warm shower, or use a hot water bottle for a few minutes before you exercise.

Abdominal bracing exercise

The following exercise is referred to a number of times in the book, so it is given here in more detail (Figs 1.17–1.19). It is called 'bracing' because in this exercise the abdominal muscles are used to literally act like a 'brace' (or corset) to keep the back stable.

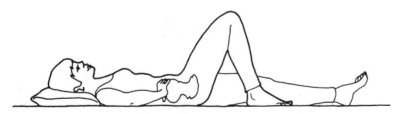

Fig. 1.17 Starting position.

Place fingers just inside the bony points of your pelvis at the front. Now draw in the low part of your tummy. If you are doing this exercise correctly, you should feel your deep abdominal muscles tightening under your thumbs. You do not have to do a maximum contraction – about half-maximum is sufficient – but try to hold the contraction for up to 20 seconds, breathing at the same time. If you have difficulty contracting the correct muscles, try imagining that you have a diamond in your tummy button and want to hide it away!

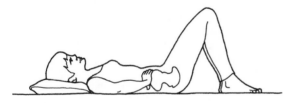

Fig. 1.18 Leg slide.

When you have mastered bracing in the starting position, try bracing and, at the same time, slide one heel along the floor, still bracing. Then bend your knee up again and relax your tummy. Repeat with the other leg, bracing first.

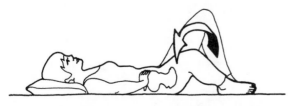

Fig. 1.19 Knee lowering.

The next progression is bracing and then, at the same time, *slowly* lowering one knee down to one side without twisting your back. Make sure you don't lift your hip up on the opposite side while you do this. Now slowly bring the knee back and relax. Repeat with the opposite knee, bracing first.

The starting position for this exercise is lying down with the knees bent up (as in Fig. 1.17). This is usually the easiest position in which to get the abdominal muscles to contract. However, it is important that we also brace our abdominal muscles to protect our backs while we move from one position to another, for example getting up from sitting down, reaching upwards, lifting etc. Thus it is particularly useful when we learn to progress from the starting position to bracing in other positions. Try bracing when sitting down and standing. Eventually it should become automatic for you to brace when moving from one position to another.

2
Causes of back pain and self-help

How to identify your problem

Most back pain is not caused by serious disease. It is what is called 'mechanical': in other words, something has gone wrong with the mechanical working of the spine. Just as the mechanics of a car can go wrong, so can the mechanics of your spine, especially if it is used incorrectly. But, unlike the car, which comes with its own manual, the spine comes with no instructions on how to use it! Nowadays our bodies are expected to cope with situations that they are not equipped to cope with, such as sitting on chairs for long periods when working with computers, being cramped up in cars or walking on hard, unyielding pavements. Fortunately for us, however, the body has an in-built capacity to heal itself, given the chance, and provided the damage is not too severe.

Your problem may be that you feel discomfort, a slight ache or you may have sharp pain, sometimes spreading into your arm(s) or leg(s). If this is the first time you have had this problem, you can be assured that, no matter how bad the pain is, it is likely to be self-limiting, *providing you take appropriate action.*

This chapter deals with the most common causes of back pain, which have been grouped into 'syndromes', and gives advice on how to deal with them. You will see that the advice for each person varies depending on what is wrong with your back or neck, so first read the description of each syndrome to see which of the symptoms (i.e. what is felt) are similar to yours. Then, having identified the syndrome which sounds like your own problem, read on to see what you can do to help it. Syndromes are not always clear cut because the shape of our spines and amount of suppleness varies from person to person, so to get a clearer overall picture, also read the next chapter on 'Posture' and any other chapters which apply to you. If you are still in any doubt about your problem, do seek the help of a chartered physiotherapist (*see* address on p. 96).

Syndrome 1: Back strain

Description

This is the most common cause of backache which is often referred to as a 'postural' ache. It comes on *gradually*, often over months or years, and can occur at any age. Back strain is due to keeping the back in one position (usually bent forwards) for too long (Fig. 2.1). The ligaments become over-stretched and start to ache; then the muscles tighten up as a reflex mechanism, causing a feeling of stiffness in the back. Aching is usually nature's way of warning you that further stretching in a bent position will lead to damage (Fig. 2.2).

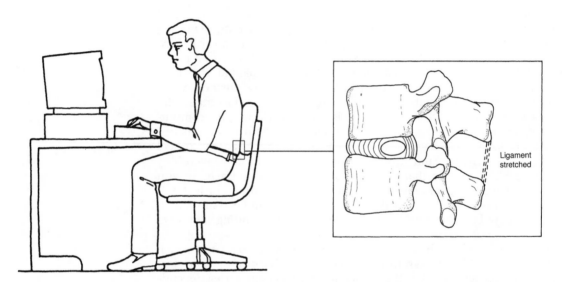

Ligament stretched

Fig. 2.1 Poor sitting posture.

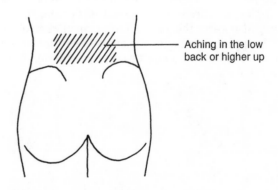

Aching in the low back or higher up

Fig. 2.2 Where the ache is felt.

What you feel

- You will feel aching in the back or neck after bending over for too long or after sitting slouched.
- The back may feel tight.
- In the early stages of this syndrome, the ache is eased by changing position.
- In the later stages, the ache may persist until you lie down, and then prevent you from getting off to sleep.
- Your back feels better after a night's rest.

Self-help

- Correct your standing and sitting posture (*see* pp. 62 and 56).
- Make sure your furniture is the correct height for you (*see* p. 58), especially if you are taller or smaller than average.
- Change your position frequently *before* the aching starts.

Interrupt long periods of sitting or bending by standing and leaning backwards and by walking. Go for a walk in your lunch-break – swing your arms to give your back some gentle movement. Do some form of exercise you enjoy that safely exercises the back, such as swimming.

Exercises

Figures 2.3–2.5 show some suitable exercises for combating back strain.

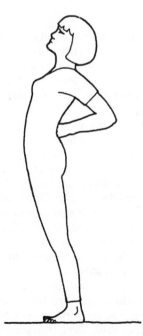

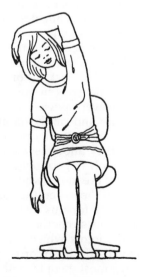

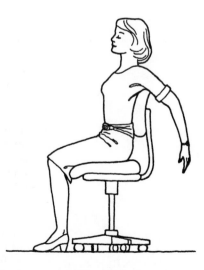

Fig. 2.3 Stand with your feet slightly apart. Push hips forwards, then lean backwards.

Fig. 2.4 Alternately stretch each side.

Fig. 2.5 Stretch backwards over edge of backrest.

Loose ligaments (hypermobility)

Description

The correct name for this condition is 'hypermobility' (hyper = too much). Some people are born with ligaments that are looser than normal, causing them to be more supple than average (Figs 2.6–2.8). They are sometimes referred to as being 'double-jointed' but this is a misnomer because the joints are perfectly normal, apart from their excessive mobility. We now know that hypermobility is responsible for many of the aches and pains that some extra-supple people suffer from. Interestingly, these people

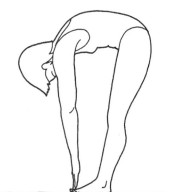

Fig. 2.6 Normal mobility.

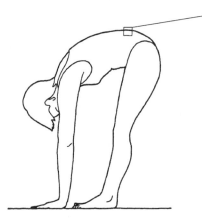

Fig. 2.7 Excessive mobility.

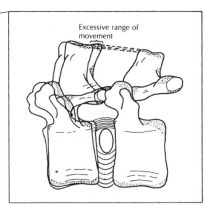

Fig. 2.8

often do not realize that they are extra-supple as their movements feel normal to them; but in fact, when their joints stiffen up in the slightest they feel very stiff. Hypermobility is the most common cause of 'growing pains' in children. While it is common knowledge that stiff joints can cause problems, symptoms related to hypermobility are only just being recognized by some people in the medical profession.

Hypermobility is usually inherited: all the joints in the body can be affected (*see* Fig. 2.9) or just one or two. It has its advantages in that many hypermobile people excel in athletics or ballet, making full use of their suppleness. However, as well as the ligaments being longer, they also tend to be weaker and can be strained more easily. Normal 'tight' ligaments keep the joints stable, protecting them, but if the ligaments are long and weak they allow *too much* movement in the spinal joints. This is why people with hypermobility often complain that their balance is poor – their joints are more 'wobbly'. Often the wrong muscles try to stabilize the joints. If, however, the correct muscles are well toned-up, they can often make up for this instability and, therefore, specific exercises which stabilize and strengthen the spine play an important part in the self-help regime. Joints which are in good alignment are less likely to suffer from any ill-effects, so correct posture is also important (*see* Chapter 3). Fortunately, most people with hypermobility have no symptoms at all.

Because of hormonal changes, the ligaments become even looser during pregnancy and for up to 6 months after the birth, and they are par-

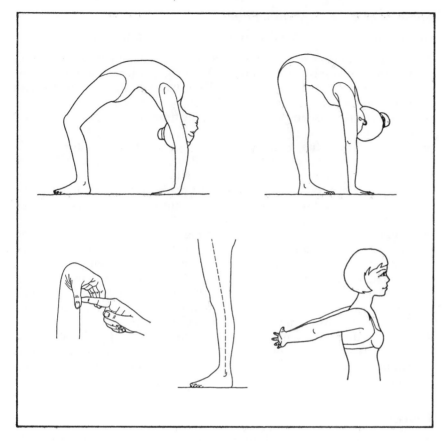

Fig. 2.9 Generalized joint hypermobility: excessive movements can be exhibited in many joints.

ticularly at risk during this period. The sacroiliac joint ligaments are particularly vulnerable during this time (*see* p. 80).

Often people with hypermobility have flat feet because the loose ligaments have caused the arches to drop, and this causes the feet and legs to roll inwards: this has a knock-on effect on the back, often causing it to be too hollow.

Symptoms

- Children tend to get aching legs after exercise, often in bed at night. This sometimes keeps them awake.
- The area between the shoulder blades may become painful if it starts to stiffen up. This is one of the first areas to give symptoms in young women.
- Low backache can occur when standing for long periods; this is eased by sitting, though people with hypermobility often fidget a lot when sitting and tend to choose positions that other people would find uncomfortable (Fig. 2.10).
- The low backache is usually worse during menstruation.

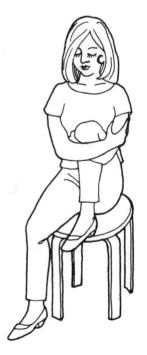

Fig. 2.10 A typical sitting posture for someone with hypermobility.

Self-help

Often a number of joints have to be taken into consideration.

- Avoid prolonged stretching of any joint, especially when any kind of weight is involved. For example, don't carry a heavy bag with your elbow straight; it is better to hold the bag next to your body with your elbow *bent*.
- Never bend, twist and lift all at the same time. *See* pp. 67–71 for advice on lifting.
- If your feet are flat, wear shoes with a good support under the arch or, better still, use special insoles called orthotics in your shoes (*see* p. 64) to help your posture and relieve backache.
- Adults with hypermobility appear to be more prone to hand, wrist and arm pain following repetitive use of the mouse or keyboard when working at a visual display unit.
- If your knees bend backwards (*see* Fig. 2.9), be careful not to stand like this; apart from straining the ligaments in your knees, it also makes your back arch too much. When you stand, bend your knees just a small amount; they will feel a bit wobbly at first because you are making your thigh muscles work. *See* p. 62 for further advice on posture when standing. When you walk, don't let your knees lock backwards – every time they do, it will jar your back.
- For care during pregnancy and after childbirth *see* pp. 79–86.
- Aerobics is *bad* for people with this condition if they do not have good alignment (*see* p. 65): sooner or later people damage themselves. Tai Chi is much safer and better for your joints.

Exercises

- Swimming is usually helpful because it tones up the muscles without weight going through the joints. However, you may find that the breast-stroke strains your back and neck if you do not swim with your face down in the water. The crawl or back-stroke may be better for you.
- Even though your ligaments are extra long, they will benefit from *gentle* stretching, provided this is done in the right way. Don't prolong a stretch because this could damage the ligaments: intermittent stretching is much better, i.e. gently stretch out the joints and then immediately release the stretch.
- Try the stretches shown in Figs 2.11–2.15 to see if they give you relief.

The 'pelvic tilting' exercises shown in Figs 2.16–2.18 will help keep your low back supple. When your pelvis moves, so does your low back. These exercises are particularly useful if your back is aching.

Stretching alone, however, will not give you a strong back. It is also essential that you learn to *stabilize* your low back by bracing (tensing) your deep abdominal muscles (Fig. 2.19). Progressions of this exercise are shown on p. 7. They should be done carefully and accurately. Learn to 'brace' during everyday activities such as getting out of a chair, leaning over the sink, bending down and rising from bending and it will become second nature to you. Strengthening your gluteal muscles (buttocks) will also help, *see* Fig. 2.55 on p. 27.

It is also important to realize that some exercises strain the neck and low back (*see*, for example, Fig. 2.20).

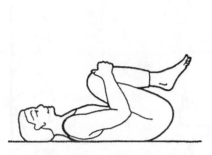

Fig. 2.11 Bend both knees up to your chest. If you still don't feel a stretch in your low back, putting a lever-arch file or a cushion under your buttocks will stretch it more.

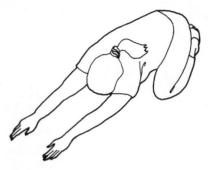

Fig. 2.12 This is a good stretch for the whole of your back.

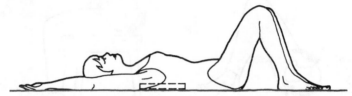

Fig. 2.13 This is a good stretch for the area between your shoulder blades. Place the folded newspaper or firm pad so that it ends at the area where you get symptoms for maximum effect.

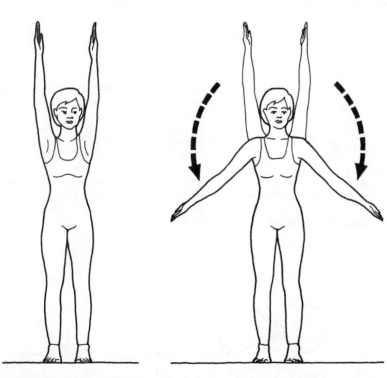

Fig. 2.14 Stretch up both arms, stretching the whole of your spine at the same time.

Fig. 2.15 Keeping your spine stretched, slowly lower your arms.

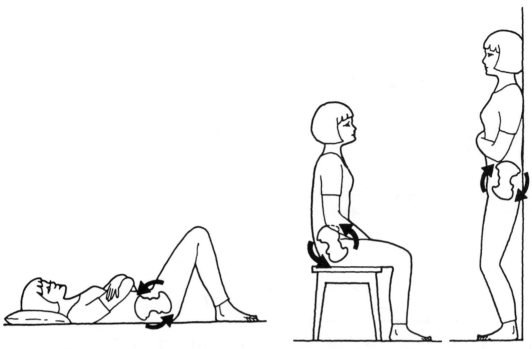

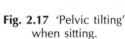

Fig. 2.16 'Pelvic tilting' exercise. Push your low back down into the floor. Hold for 10 seconds, then relax.

Fig. 2.17 'Pelvic tilting' when sitting.

Fig. 2.18 'Pelvic tilting' when standing.

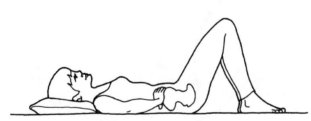

Fig. 2.19 Stabilization exercise: abdominal 'bracing'.

Place fingers just inside the bony points of your pelvis at the front. Now draw in the low part of your tummy: this is called 'bracing'. If you are doing this exercise correctly, you should feel your deep abdominal muscles tightening under your thumbs. You do not have to do a maximum contraction – about half-maximum is sufficient – but try to hold the contraction for up to 20 seconds, breathing at the same time. If you have difficulty contracting the correct muscles, try imagining that you have a diamond in your tummy button and want to hide it away!

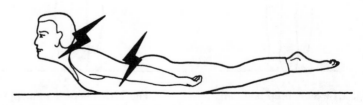

Fig. 2.20 Hyperextension. This exercise is bad for both your back and neck.

Syndrome 2: Disc problems

Disc tear/bulge

The functions of the discs are to absorb jolts from the legs when you walk, run or jump, and to cushion the weight that goes through them (even just your body weight). They also allow movement between the vertebrae. Disc problems often occur in the most flexible areas of the spine, for example at the bottom of it, or in the middle of your neck. The weakest part of the disc is the back part, usually to one side (*see* Fig. 2.22). Refer back to pp. 1–4 for information on the structure of the discs.

Minor disc problems are common and occur even in teenagers, but they can lead to more serious problems if the right precautions are not taken. The symptoms people get from disc problems vary according to which stage the damaged disc has reached (Figs 2.21–2.25).

Description

Although a disc can tear suddenly because of an accident such as a fall, the most common cause of damage is *repeated minor injuries over many years due to awkward bending and lifting* (*see* Fig. 1.10 on p. 4). Often the

Progression of disc problems

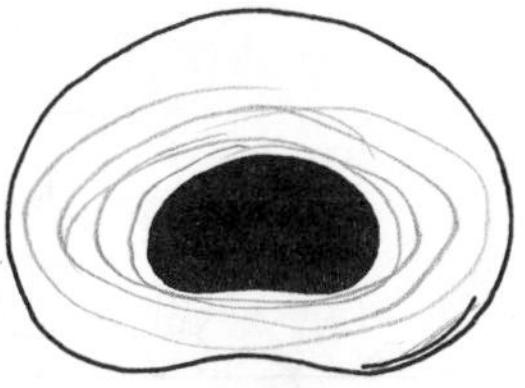

Fig. 2.22 Disruption of fibres at back of disc.

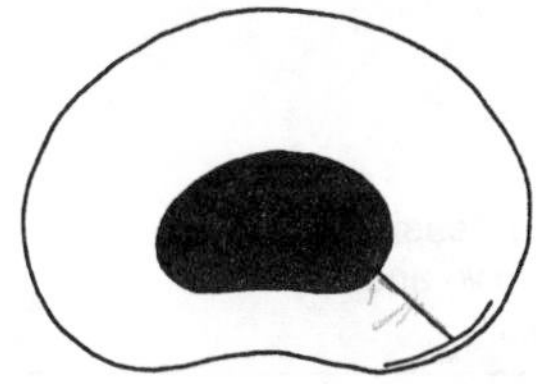

Fig. 2.23 Tears in annular part of disc. Once this has occurred, the nucleus gradually becomes more like crab meat than a gel!

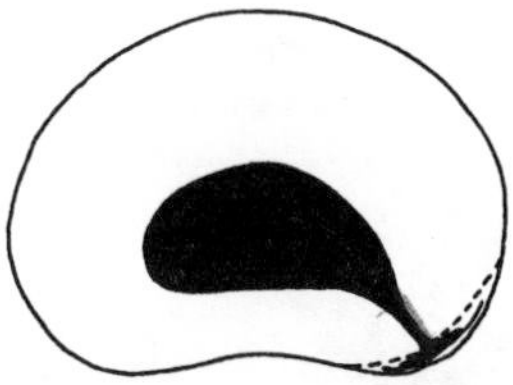

Fig. 2.24 Bulging disc. The nucleus – or fragments of it – travels down one of these tears. (This is often referred to as a 'slipped disc', but in fact the disc itself does not 'slip'; rather a fragment of the nucleus moves within the disc.)

THE AIM IS TO STOP THIS PROGRESSION

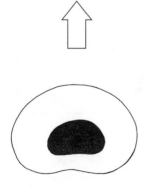

Fig. 2.21 A healthy disc.

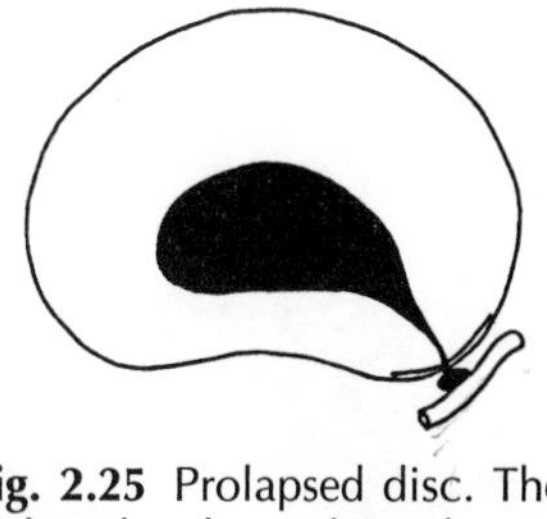

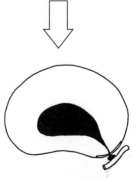

Fig. 2.25 Prolapsed disc. The nucleus has burst through outer annulus and is pressing on a nerve causing 'sciatica' (pain in the leg).

damage *appears* to have been caused by a trivial incident such as reaching forwards to lift something quite light, but in fact this is often the 'last straw'. The disc may have been torn previously and just caused slight aching in the low back, which may have been thought to be 'muscular'.

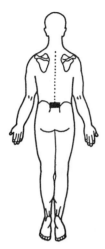

Fig. 2.26 Initially there may be central low back pain or discomfort.

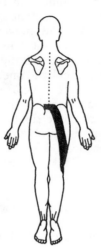

Fig. 2.27 Later the pain spreads into the leg.

Fig. 2.28a It may be difficult for you to straighten your back.

Fig. 2.28b Some people are 'windswept' over to one side.

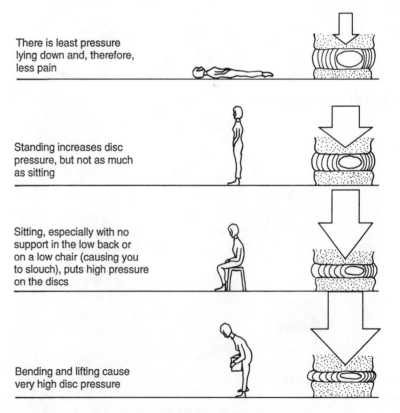

There is least pressure lying down and, therefore, less pain

Standing increases disc pressure, but not as much as sitting

Sitting, especially with no support in the low back or on a low chair (causing you to slouch), puts high pressure on the discs

Bending and lifting cause very high disc pressure

Fig. 2.29 Pressure on the disc.

Symptoms

These may come on suddenly or gradually over several hours or days, and the location and severity of the pain can vary (Figs 2.26, 2.27).

- The pain is made worse by bending forwards.
- The pain may either be eased by leaning backwards, or made worse if you lean too far backwards.
- Your back may be straight or you may be bent forwards (Fig. 2.28a). Some people's shoulders are shifted over to one side in relation to their hips (Fig. 2.28b), giving them the feeling that something is 'out of place'. This can either be due to muscle spasm or to movement of a fragment of the nucleus within the disc.
- The pain is worse in some positions which cause increased pressure on the disc (Fig. 2.29).
- The exercises shown in Figs 2.30 and 2.31 are bad for you because they increase disc pressure a lot.

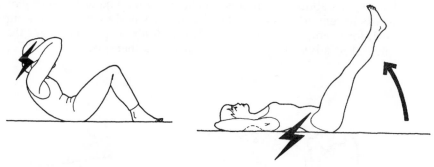

Fig. 2.30 Sit-ups.   **Fig. 2.31** Double leg lifts.

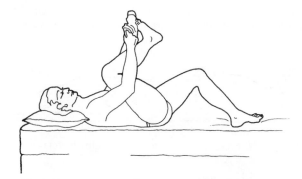

Fig. 2.32 Put on your socks or tights lying down.

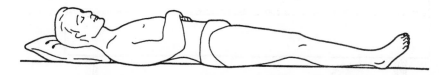

Fig. 2.33 Lying straight arches the back slightly, especially
if the surface you are lying on is very firm.

Self-help

- 'Controlled activity' is necessary for a while; in other words, you should cut down on activities and postures which increase disc pressure until your symptoms ease off. This may take a day or two, or several weeks.
- Only if the pain is severe and all movements painful should you resort to complete bedrest (*see* p. 73).
- Don't bend your back in the early stages: this would prevent it from healing (*see* Fig. 2.32).
- Stand or walk rather than sit.
- Give your back a rest for periods during the day, choosing whichever of the resting positions shown in Figs 2.33–2.35 is most comfortable for you.
- If your bed is too soft, get someone to put 2 cm chipboard under your mattress to make it firmer (Fig. 2.36). Don't sleep on a hard floor – you would find it impossible to relax.
- A temporary corset or sports belt (which can be purchased from your local sports shop or sometimes a chemists) may be useful for *up to* 3 weeks to remind you not to bend your back and to give it some support, for example when travelling. But don't keep it on longer than this unless advised to do so by your physiotherapist.

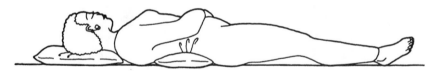

Fig. 2.34 A cushion or rolled up towel under the low back arches it more. Some people find they need to add an extra pillow under the head for comfort.

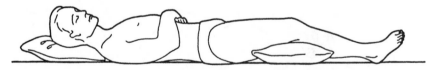

Fig. 2.35 One or two pillows under your knees helps to relax your low back.

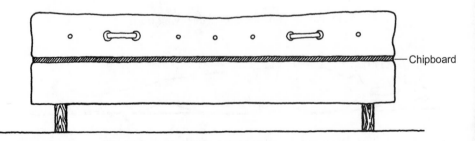

Fig. 2.36 How to make a bed firmer.

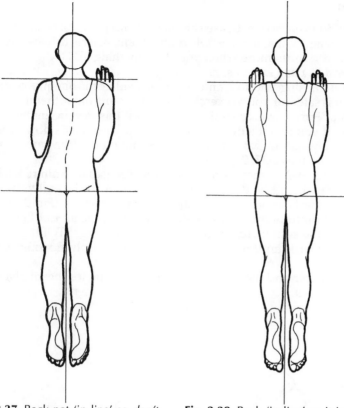

Fig. 2.37 Back not 'in line' so *don't* do any exercises until you have straightened it up.

Fig. 2.38 Back 'in line' so it is safe to proceed with the next exercise.

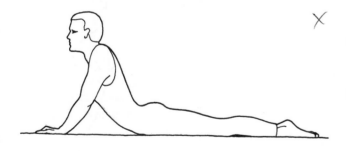

Fig. 2.39 Push up with your arms, keeping your hips down, and let your low back sag into an arch, then lower the top half of your body down again. (Adapted from R.A. McKenzie, 1981. *The Lumbar Spine: Mechanical Diagnosis and Therapy.* Spinal Publications.) Make sure your back is 'in line' first (*see* Figs 2.37, 2.38). If your back is acutely painful, it may be more effective to sustain this position for a minute or two before lowering your body very slowly.

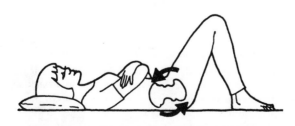

Fig. 2.40 'Pelvic tilting': gently flatten your low back against the floor and then make it hollow.

Exercises

- Only do exercises that ease the pain. If the pain starts spreading or increasing in intensity, STOP doing them. Learn to listen to your body: if it hurts more when you do something, STOP.
- *Before doing any exercises, make sure your back is 'in line'.* If your back pain is causing you to lean over to one side or if one hip is sticking out, it is safer for you to exercise lying on your front rather than standing up. First move your hips across until they are in line with your body. If you're not sure that they are, put your hands down the side of your waist to make sure it feels symmetrical (the same on both sides) (*see* Figs 2.37, 2.38).
- Figures 2.39–2.42 show some extension exercises for pain relief. These exercises should be done 10 times each hour in the early stages – it is particularly important to do the 'extension exercise' (Fig. 2.41) when you get up from the sitting position. They are meant to REDUCE the pain. If the pain increases or spreads into the leg, STOP!
- As your back improves, try swimming, or simply floating on your back.
- Some people find that hanging while holding on to a beam gives temporary relief.

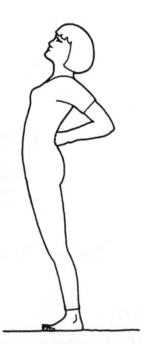 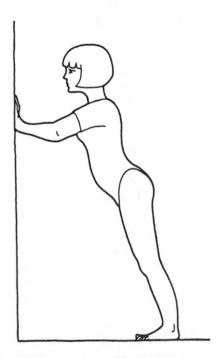

Fig. 2.41 Extension exercise. Stand with your feet slightly apart. Push your hips forwards, then lean backwards. This exercise can also be done with your buttocks resting against a table for support – then lean backwards over the table.

Fig. 2.42 Support your hands on a wall. Let your low back sag into an arch.

Sitting

This is usually the biggest problem – only start to sit if it does not induce pain. Don't bend your back when you sit in the early stages. Try one or two of the suggestions shown in Figs 2.43–2.45. Figures 2.46–2.48 relate to rising from sitting.

Other problem areas

- **Driving** puts very high pressure on your back (*see* p. 59).
- **Lifting**: *Don't* until the pain is less, otherwise it could return with a vengeance.

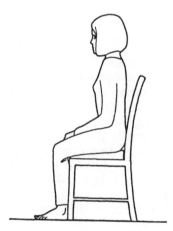

Fig. 2.43 Sitting on a posture wedge with your knees below your hips reduces disc pressure.

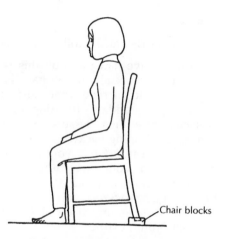

Chair blocks

Fig. 2.44 Blocks under the back legs of your chair have the same effect.

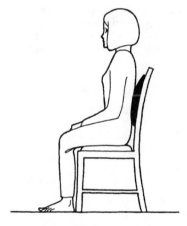

Fig. 2.45 A backrest or cushion behind your low back helps to straighten it.

Rising from sitting

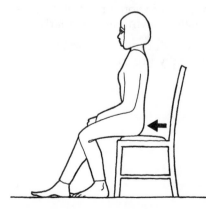

Fig. 2.46 Slide forwards to the edge of the chair: armrests help.

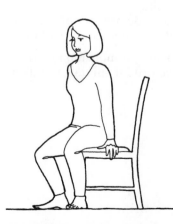

Fig. 2.47 Turn your body to whichever side is most comfortable, avoiding twisting your back.

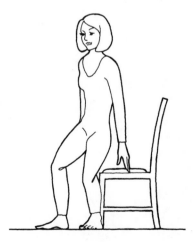

Fig. 2.48 Now straighten your knees.

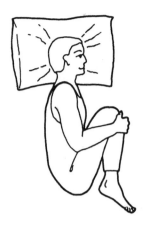

Fig. 2.49 Bend up your knees until you feel a *gentle* stretch in your low back, but don't go any further if it is painful.

- **When to start bending**: When you can sit for an hour with no ill-effect, try gently bending your back when lying on whichever side is more comfortable – don't go too far to begin with and always straighten your back immediately afterwards. Then, over a period of 3 weeks, see if you can gradually increase the bending until you are able to bend as shown in Fig. 2.49.
- **Preventing recurrences**: This type of back problem is fairly unique in that the pain may be severe on one day and gone the next. It is, therefore, tempting to think that everything is back to normal and to act accordingly. However, this is not the case. The pain goes well before healing is complete, so it is important that you learn to use your back correctly.

Risk times

Your back is at risk at the following times:

1. After you have had the 'flu': this tends to 'weaken' the back for a week or so, especially if you have had to rest in bed with it.
2. If you have to sit more than normal or on poor seats, for example travelling on holiday, attending a conference or sitting on low sofas at social gatherings. Be sure to interrupt long periods of sitting by getting up, leaning backwards and walking about a little. If you need to bend forwards while you are sitting down, get into the habit of bending from your hips rather than your back (i.e. bend from the groin area, not from round the waist). You may have to take a posture wedge or backrest with you to meetings if you do not know what the chairs are going to be like. Avoid low sofas at all costs – *see* Chapter 3 on 'Posture'.
3. If you have to sleep in a saggy bed, for example on holiday, give advance warning to hotels that you need a firm or medium-firm bed. If this doesn't work, there is usually room to put a single mattress on the floor.
4. With repetitive heavy lifting; so be sure to read the section in Chapter 3 on 'Lifting', and learn to brace your deep abdominal muscles before you lift.
5. When you are 'out of condition'. Take part in some form of exercise that does not jerk or jar your back, such as swimming regularly.

Often it is a combination of risk factors which causes the problem, for example driving all day and then lifting heavy luggage.

Prolapsed disc causing 'trapped nerve' (sciatica)

Description

When a disc 'prolapses', the inner part of it, the nucleus, escapes through a tear in the outer part of the disc (the annulus), and starts to press on whichever nerve is next to it. This causes pain in the leg, called 'sciatica', which usually spreads below the knee. (The sciatic nerve is one of the main nerves in the leg.) It is commonly referred to as a 'trapped nerve'.

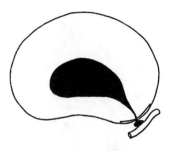

Fig. 2.50 A prolapsed disc.

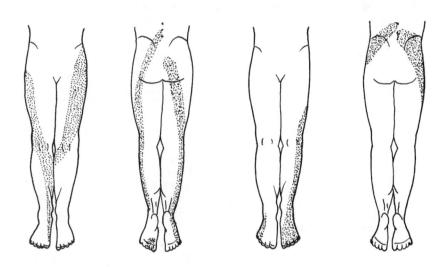

Fig. 2.51 Most common areas of pain. Depending on which nerve is affected, pain is felt in all or part of one of these areas.

Symptoms

Symptoms are now very different from when the disc was just torn.

- Pain is now more severe, spreading into the leg, usually below the knee, but it may be less in the back. Occasionally there is no back pain at all.
- Either immediately, or over the course of the next 3 weeks, *neurological signs* may develop, showing that the adjacent nerve is being irritated or compressed. 'Pins and needles' may be felt first of all. More serious signs are numbness (or 'deadness') in an area of the skin in the leg and/or weakness of the muscles in the foot or leg. The ankle or knee jerk may be absent.
- It is difficult to find a comfortable position, and rest does not provide much relief.
- Walking makes the pain worse.
- Sitting makes the pain worse after a while and it is more comfortable with the weight on one side to take the pressure off the affected buttock/leg.
- Coughing or sneezing may make the pain shoot into the leg.
- *NB If your bladder function is affected, i.e. if you are unable to pass water or to control urination, this is an emergency: contact your doctor immediately.*

Self-help/treatment

- If you are in severe pain, you should ask your doctor to visit you at home. You will be prescribed pain-relieving tablets and may be referred for a consultation with an orthopaedic surgeon, rheumatologist or a chartered physiotherapist.
- Try and discover comfortable resting positions (*see* Figs 2.52, 2.53). Once the disc has prolapsed, self-help is difficult in the early stages as there may be no single position which provides pain relief for long. Moving to a different position eases the pain for a while. A hard bed is usually more comfortable as it is easier to move in – *see* pp. 73–77 concerning 'bedrest'.

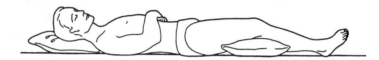

Fig. 2.53 This position may provide pain relief for a while.

- Treatment by a physiotherapist will consist of either gentle mobilization, electrical treatment (which is not painful) to reduce the muscle spasm, or traction. Some physiotherapists are able to offer acupuncture for pain relief.
- Neurological signs such as 'deadness' (numbness), weakness or tingling should be monitored by a physiotherapist or doctor because, if they get worse, surgery may be indicated.
- Following an episode such as this, even if the symptoms have reduced considerably, attention to correct posture and lifting (*see* pp. 49–71) is essential, and repetitive heavy lifting is inadvisable.
- Attending a back education programme or back school is useful to help you regain confidence and build up the strength of your muscles. Your doctor or physiotherapist will be able to advise you about this.

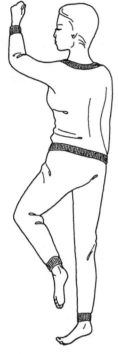

Fig. 2.52 Modified prone-lying position. This position may provide pain relief for a while.

Exercises

- Any exercises which cause pain either at the time or the next day should be avoided. There is, understandably, a tendency for people not to want to move their backs at all after such a severe bout of pain. However, ending up with a rigid back can cause problems by forcing another part of the body to take the strain, so it is important to regain some mobility. It is better to avoid *extremes* of bending forwards or leaning backwards for long periods.
- Later on, exercises should be aimed at strengthening the deep abdominal (tummy) muscles, in particular, and the muscles in the buttocks (the gluteal muscles), and stretching the hamstring muscles behind the back of the thighs.

Abdominal bracing exercises

These help to stabilize the low back and prevent unwanted movement. Figure 2.54 illustrates this exercise. For a progression of this exercise, *see*

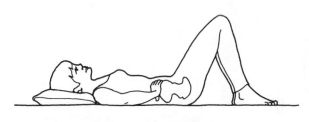

Fig. 2.54 Abdominal bracing exercise.

Place your fingers just inside the bony points of your pelvis at the front. Now draw in the low part of your tummy: this is called 'bracing'. If you are doing this exercise correctly, you should feel your deep abdominal muscles tightening under your thumbs. You do not have to do a maximum contraction – about half-maximum is sufficient – but try to hold the contraction for up to 20 seconds, breathing at the same time. If you have difficulty contracting the correct muscles, try imagining that you have a diamond in your tummy button and want to hide it away!

Figs 1.18–1.19. Get into the habit of bracing your deep abdominal muscles whenever you stretch up your arms, lift etc. to protect your back.

Gluteal muscle strengthening

When the gluteal muscles (your buttocks) are strong, they take some of the load off the back muscles when you walk and lift. Figure 2.55 illustrates this exercise.

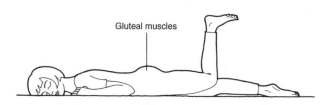

Gluteal muscles

Fig. 2.55 Gluteal muscle strengthening. Some people find it more comfortable to have a pillow under tummy.

First brace your deep abdominal muscles (*see* Fig. 2.54), then bend one knee and lift this leg up a little – don't arch your low back. Now lower this leg, straighten the knee and relax your abdominal muscles. Repeat with the other leg, bracing first.

Hamstring stretches

You have to be careful with hamstring stretches that you do not cause sciatica, so do not do these stretches in the early stages while you still have leg pain. Then, when you stretch your hamstrings, make sure you keep the back straight and apply the stretch very gradually. Figures 2.56a and b illustrate this exercise.

Forecast

- Symptoms often die down gradually, but in more severe cases it can take up to 18 months for this to occur.
- If neurological symptoms worsen, then surgery may be indicated.

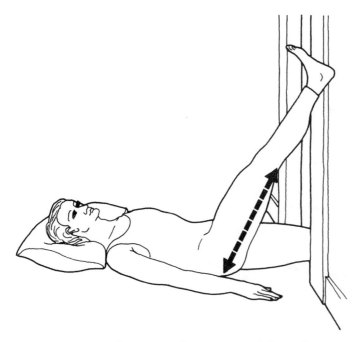

Keeping your right knee straight, slowly slide your right foot up the wall until you feel a slight stretch at the back of your thigh above your knee. Hold for 20 seconds, then bend your knee to take off the stretch.

Fig. 2.56a Safe way to stretch hamstrings.

Put one foot on a ledge or stool – a low one to start with – and, keeping your knee straight, bend forwards from the *hip* (not the back, which should be kept straight) until you feel a slight stretch at the back of your thigh above your knee. Hold for 20 seconds, then bend your knee to take off the stretch.

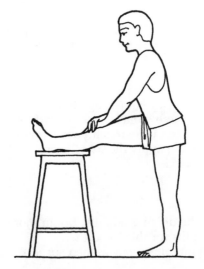

Fig. 2.56b A more advanced hamstring stretch.

Syndrome 3: Facet joint problems

Description

The facet joints are small joints on each side of the spine (Figs 2.57, 2.58). As we get older, some 'wear and tear' in these joints often occurs but it does not necessarily cause pain. However, the joints can become painful if *too much stress* goes through them when: (a) the back is too hollow – this makes the back muscles tighten up, squashing the facet joints (Figs 2.59, 2.60); or (b) if the disc between the facet joints has been narrowed due to previous damage (Fig. 2.61).

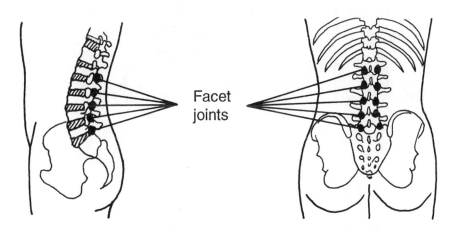

Facet
joints

Fig. 2.57 Side view of low back.   **Fig. 2.58** Back view of low back.

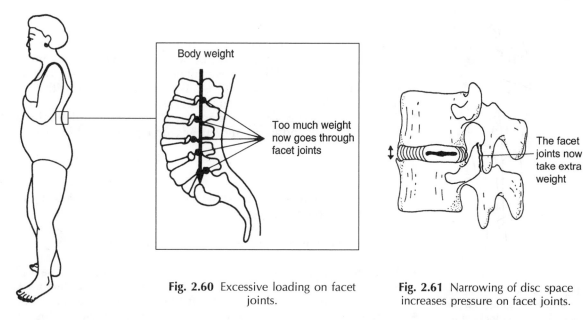

Body weight

Too much weight
now goes through
facet joints

The facet
joints now
take extra
weight

Fig. 2.60 Excessive loading on facet
joints.

Fig. 2.61 Narrowing of disc space
increases pressure on facet joints.

Fig. 2.59 Hollow back.

Where the pain is felt

Depending on which joint/s are affected, you will feel a deep ache or pain either over the joint/s themselves or at some distance from them: this is called *referred* pain (*see* Fig. 2.62).

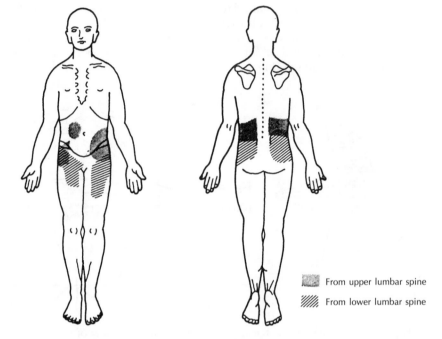

From upper lumbar spine

From lower lumbar spine

Fig. 2.62 Areas of 'referred' pain from facet joints in the lumbar spine (low back).

Symptoms

- The ache/pain is made worse by: standing still for long periods, bending backwards, reaching upwards, walking slowly or for long distances, leaning (e.g. doing the washing-up), wearing shoes with heels over 4 cm (2 inches) high, cold weather, wearing shoes with *too low* a heel and sleeping on your tummy (Fig. 2.63).
- The ache/pain is *eased* by: sitting (for short periods), flattening the low back (i.e. rounding it) and curling up on your side in bed.

Self-help

- **Pain relief positions** are those which flatten your low back. It is not helpful to go on bedrest as this would make your back stiffen up, but try giving your back some relief for one or two 15-minute periods during the day in whichever of the positions shown in Figs 2.64–2.66 help.
- **Your bed**: A bed which is *too firm* can make the pain worse. Often the ideal surface is one which is medium-firm, for example a pocket-sprung mattress (*see* pp. 49–53 for further advice on beds).
- **How to stand correctly**: First turn to pp. 61–64 for advice on the effect of footwear and orthotics (insoles) on your back, and on the best way

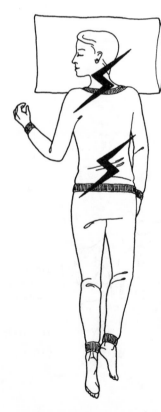

Fig. 2.63 DON'T sleep on your tummy as this arches your low back, locking up the facet joints.

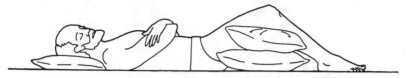

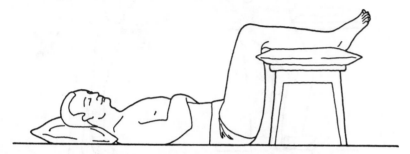

Fig. 2.64 Here the spine is bent more, which suits people with facet joint problems.

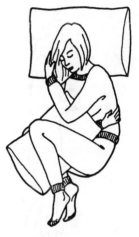

Fig. 2.66 Lying on your side (with the painful side uppermost) is often the preferred position for sleeping.

Fig. 2.65 As above, the spine is bent more in this position.

to stand. Your back will tend to arch too much when you reach upwards (Fig. 2.67) or lean forwards, for example over a sink. To prevent this, first flatten your low back by 'pelvic tilting' as shown in Fig. 2.68 (*see* p. 16 and Fig. 2.18 also). Standing still for long periods tends to make the back stiffen up. Try to prevent this by following the advice illustrated in Figs 2.69–2.71.

● **How to sit correctly**: Learn how to sit correctly in a position that suits

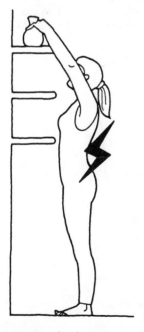

Fig. 2.67 Low back tends to arch when reaching upwards.

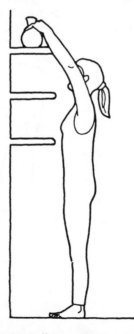

Fig. 2.68 Pull in your tummy muscles to flatten your low back (i.e. 'pelvic tilt') as you reach upwards.

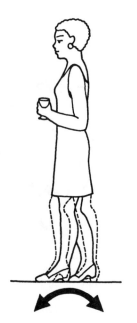

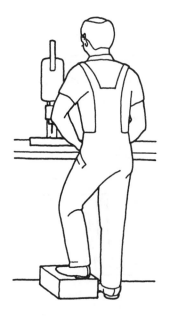

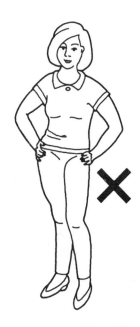

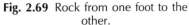

Fig. 2.69 Rock from one foot to the other.

Fig. 2.70 Put one foot up on a block.

Fig. 2.71 DON'T habitually stand lopsided like this!

your back (*see* p. 56). Don't be tempted to 'sit up straight' in a rigid way as this may over-arch your low back. Although sitting for short periods relieves your back pain, after a while you probably get uncomfortable and start to fidget. This is because the facet joints need gentle movement. If you have no choice but to sit for a long time, for example as a passenger in a car, 'unlock' your facet joints with the exercise shown in Fig. 2.72 or by 'pelvic tilting' (*see* Fig. 2.17 on p. 16).

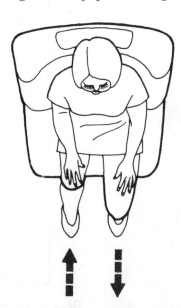

Fig. 2.72 An exercise to do to interrupt long periods of sitting in the car. Alternately push one thigh forwards, then the other.

Using backrests and footstools can help facet joint problems (Fig. 2.73), while a kneeling stool can be unhelpful (Fig. 2.74). Figure 2.75 illustrates something else which is unhelpful to the back.

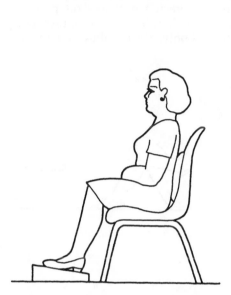 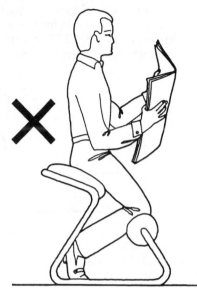

Fig. 2.73 A backrest and footstool help facet joint problems. Push your back *into* the backrest; don't arch away from it.

Fig. 2.74 A kneeling stool may be unsuitable for facet joint problems, especially if you have knee problems.

● **Lifting:** Before you lift, flatten your low back by 'pelvic tilting' (*see* Fig. 2.18). *See* pp. 67–71 for further advice on lifting. Don't bend sideways when you lift as this jams your facet joints (Fig. 2.76).

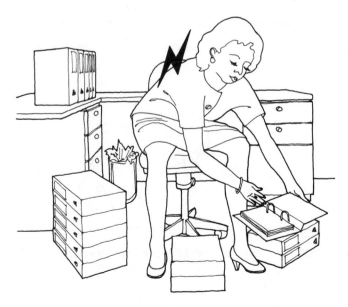 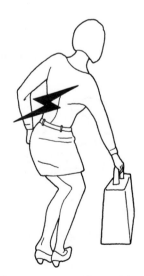

Fig. 2.75 This is NOT good for your back!

Fig. 2.76 How NOT to lift an object.

Exercises

- Usually the tummy muscles are weak with this syndrome, and exercises which flatten and strengthen the low back help. The 'pelvic tilting' exercises shown on p. 16 and bracing exercises on p. 7 are particularly suitable for this syndrome. For *early* facet joint problems, 'curl-downs' (Fig. 2.77) are useful but only *after* the above-mentioned exercises have been mastered.

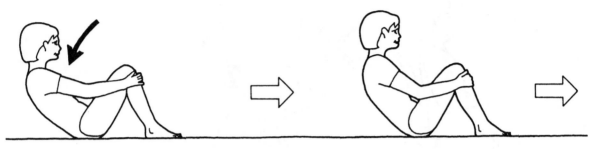

(a) Hold on to your knees. Keeping your chin in, lower your trunk slightly so that your low back flattens against the supporting surface. Hold with your hands if necessary.

(b) Lift up again to the starting position.

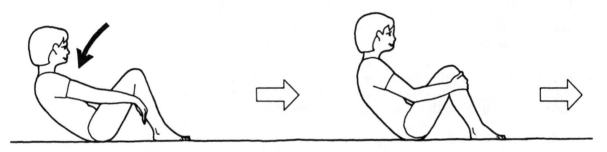

(c) Now lower your trunk slowly without using your hands. As the muscles get stronger, lower the trunk further . . .

(d) . . . always returning to the starting position.

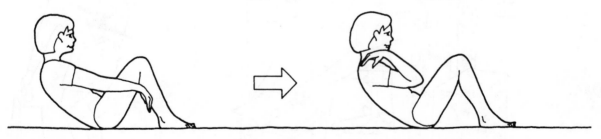

(e) Progress by statically holding a position.

(f) Then hold this position, keeping your hands on your shoulders.

Fig. 2.77 'Curl-downs'.

● Further exercises that can prove useful are those which loosen the
  back (Fig. 2.78) and those which stretch the hip muscles (Fig. 2.79).

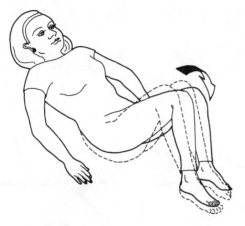

Keeping your knees together, slowly roll them
over to one side, then the other. If your back pain
is on one side of your back, only roll *away from*
the painful side for relief. This is a good exercise
to do first thing in the morning if your back feels
stiff.

Fig. 2.78 To loosen your back.

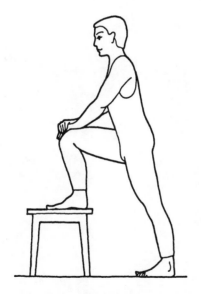

Tight hip muscles cause the back to over-arch;
to stretch them, first 'pelvic tilt' (*see* Fig. 2.18),
then lean forwards until you feel a stretch at the
front of the hip of the leg you are standing on.
Hold for 12 seconds, then relax. Repeat with the
other leg.

Fig. 2.79 A stretch for tight hip muscles.

- Exercises to strengthen the gluteal muscles in the buttocks also help this problem – *see* Fig. 2.55.
- DON'T do exercises which over-arch the back such as those shown in Figs 2.80 and 2.81.

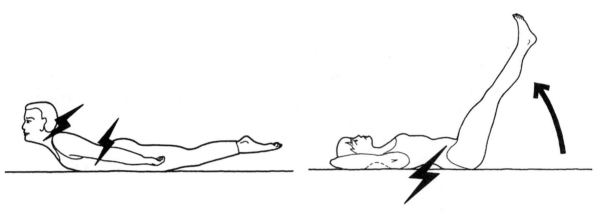

Fig. 2.80 Hyperextension.

Fig. 2.81 Double leg lifts.

Facet joint overgrowth causing 'trapped nerve' (sciatica)

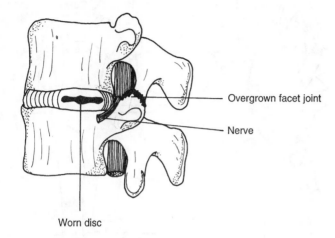

Overgrown facet joint

Nerve

Worn disc

Fig. 2.82 A second cause of sciatica.

Description

The other main cause of a nerve being 'trapped' is by an overgrowth of bone from a facet joint (Fig. 2.82). This is more common in middle-aged people, especially if they have had a lot of back pain in the past due to a disc problem.

Symptoms

- Ache or pain across the low back or to one side, and in one or both legs.
- This is eased by sitting and lying with the hips and knees bent up.
- The pain is made worse by walking.
- There may be numbness, pins and needles or weakness in the foot or leg.

Self-help

- Pain relief positions are shown in Figs 2.83–2.85.

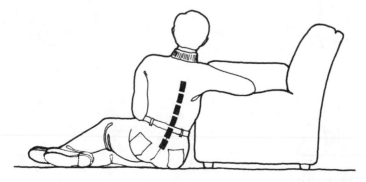

Fig. 2.83 Sit on your side with the painful side *underneath*.

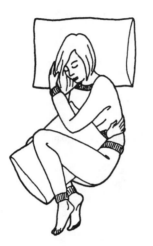

Fig. 2.84 You will be more comfortable with the painful leg on top.

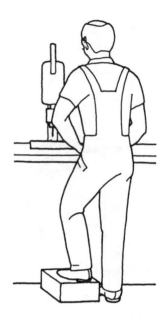

Fig. 2.85 Rest the foot of the painful leg on a block.

Exercises

- When you have pain in the leg, extreme care must be taken with exercises. Usually those which arch the back make the pain worse. Exercises to flatten the back by tightening the tummy muscles sometimes help (*see* Fig. 2.16). Figures 2.86–2.88 illustrate some further suggestions.

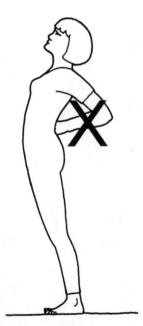

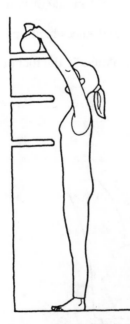

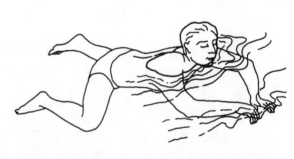

Fig. 2.88 Breaststroke done in this manner arches the back too much. Keep your face down in the water, or try the backstroke or crawl.

Fig. 2.86 Avoid arching your low back.

Fig. 2.87 Flatten your back first before reaching up.

Syndrome 4: Sacroiliac strain

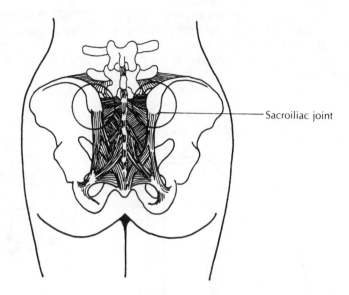

Fig. 2.89 The sacroiliac joints.

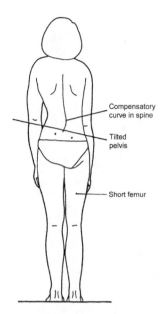

Fig. 2.90 A short leg puts a strain on the sacroiliac joints.

Description

The two sacroiliac joints join the sacrum (at the base of the spine) to the pelvis (Fig. 2.89). These joints are strong and there is very little move-ment in them. Most pain felt in the region of the sacroiliac joints origi-nates in the *spine* and not in the joints themselves, even though they may feel tender to touch. Occasionally the ligaments crossing one of the joints can be strained through a twisting movement (*see* Fig. 2.91) or a fall on the side or buttocks. The most common cause, however, is over-stretch-ing of the ligaments during, or shortly after, pregnancy.

If one leg is shorter than the other, this puts a strain on the sacroiliac joints (Fig. 2.90).

Symptoms

- Pain over one or both sacroiliac joints, and sometimes in the groin.
- This is made worse by twisting movements such as turning over in bed, getting out of a car with one leg first or stepping up on to a high stool.

Before jumping to the conclusion that you have strained your sacroiliac joint, remember that problems from the spine itself can refer pain into this area, so read Syndromes 3 and 5 to make sure of the diagnosis.

Self-help

- If you have a short leg, raising the heel of the shoe on the short side may help (*see* 'Short leg syndrome' on p. 65).
- If the pain is associated with pregnancy, use a sacroiliac binder (Fig. 5.4) and read Chapter 5 on 'Pregnancy and after childbirth'.
- 'Bracing' the deep abdominal muscles helps to stabilize the back (*see*

p. 7). Avoid stressing your joints by tightening these muscles before turning over in bed for example.

- Avoid twisting movements, for example to get out of the car; tighten your tummy muscles and lift both legs out together (and get into the car in a similar manner).
- Figures 2.91 and 2.92 give some further advice on movement and posture.

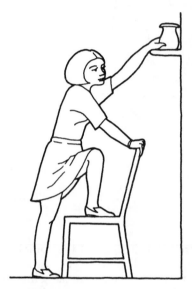

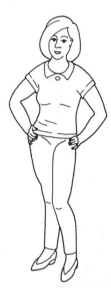

Fig. 2.91 Avoid twisting strains such as this.

Fig. 2.92 Don't stand lopsided – *see* p. 62 for advice on how to stand properly.

Syndrome 5: Neck strain

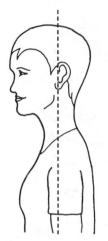
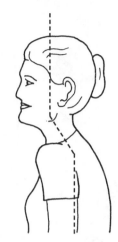

Fig. 2.93 'In line': ideal neck posture.

Fig. 2.94 'Out of line': forward head posture with rounded shoulders.

When the head is 'in line' with the rest of the body (Fig. 2.93 and cf. Fig. 2.94) the muscles at the back of the neck are relatively soft. Once the head starts to move forwards, these muscles have to work extra hard just to hold up the head, causing excessive pressure on the joints in the back of the neck. In turn, the muscles at the front of the neck become over-stretched and weak.

Common causes of neck strain and poor posture

- Figures 2.95–2.100 show some common causes of neck strain.
- Wearing bifocals: tilting the head backwards to look through the lower part of the lens can cause strain.
- Wearing spectacles with the wrong focal distance when working at a VDU: 'middle-distance' spectacles should be worn.
- Painting, especially ceilings: periodically tuck in your chin and bend the head forwards (*see* Fig. 2.104).

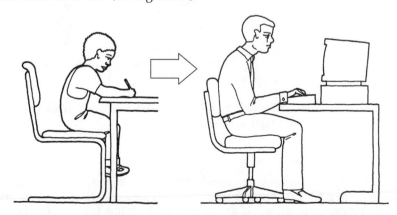

Fig. 2.95 Furniture that doesn't fit encourages this posture.

Fig. 2.96 Tense posture at work: old habits die hard.

Other common causes of neck pain and poor posture

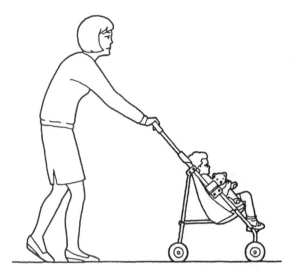

Fig. 2.97 Years of pushing prams . . .

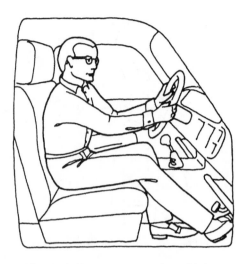

Fig. 2.98 Tense posture when driving.

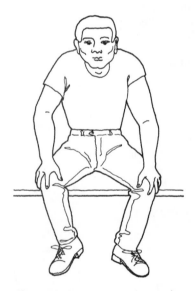

Fig. 2.99 Poor posture in youth.

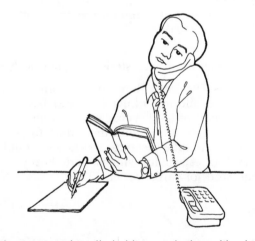

Fig. 2.100 Habitually holding a telephone like this!

- At the hairdresser's: ask to have your hair washed with your neck bent *forwards*, not backwards.

Psychological stress

Figure 2.101 shows what modern life can feel like at times – and tension aggravates neck problems in particular. If you feel that you are under constant pressure at work or home, or studying for exams, the tone in your neck muscles increases, often sufficiently to cause a recurrence of an old neck problem. Recognizing that tension plays a part in your

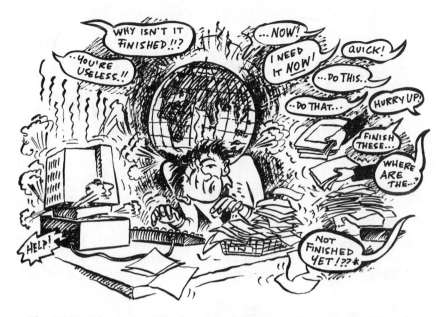

Fig. 2.101 Life can be difficult at times! (Reprinted from *Your health at the vdu: a practical guide to reducing physical stress at the workplace*, a booklet by Sheila Marks and Jean Oliver, published in 1966 by the Health Monitoring Unit Ltd. Illustration by Martin Sandhill.)

problem is the beginning of helping it, as so often people are reluctant to admit that it is, regarding tension as some kind of failure.

Tension is a large area which cannot be fully dealt with in a few lines. There may well be areas in your life that need carefully looking into, situations that need an honest appraisal. How much pressure do *you* put on yourself?

There are many different techniques which have been shown to reduce stress, such as the 'contract–relax' method of relaxation (tightening up different muscle groups in the body, then relaxing them and noting the difference) and meditation. Allowing yourself time to listen to music, or simply relaxing in a comfortable position with a heat-pad moulded round your neck will help you to cope. I would particularly recommend the booklet *Stress at work: causes, effects and prevention**. See also p. 92 for another relaxation exercise.

Symptoms

- Headaches: Most headaches are caused by tightness of muscles and joints at the nape of the neck. Aching may be felt in any of the areas shown in Fig. 2.102.
- Pain and/or stiffness in the neck itself on one or both sides.
- Muscular pain at the top of the shoulders.
- Severe joint problems in the neck can cause a 'trapped nerve' with pain in one or both arms, pins and needles, numbness and weakness.

---

* *Stress at work: causes, effects and prevention* was published by the European Foundation for the Improvement of Living and Working Conditions, 1994, and is available from HMSO Publications Centre (Tel. 0171 873 9090).

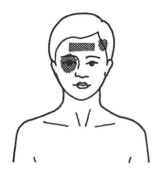
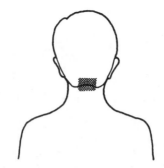
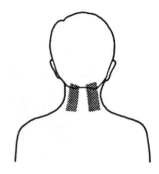

Fig. 2.102 Headaches 'referred' from the neck.

Self-help

- **Exercises** are essential to stretch the tight muscles at the back of your neck and strengthen the weak muscles at the front of the neck. Figures 2.103–2.108 show some examples.

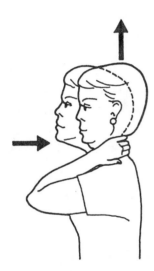

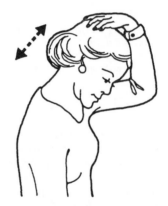

Fig. 2.104 A stretch for tight neck muscles: First tuck in your chin, then pull your head down until you can feel a stretch in the top of your neck. Hold the stretch for 12 seconds. Your chin should touch the top of your chest. If it does not, make this your aim, but it will take some weeks of gentle stretching to achieve this.

Fig. 2.103 Posture correction: Feel the muscles become softer as you tuck in your chin and lift upwards from the back of your ears.

- Your neck posture is related to the posture of your whole spine, so turn to p. 56 for how to correct your posture when sitting and p. 62 for posture correction when standing. Figures 2.109 and 2.110 show good writing posture and a writing slope, respectively.

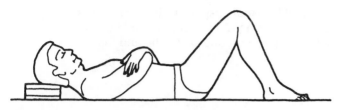

Fig. 2.105 A good stretch for the top of your neck: Lie for 10 minutes each day with your head raised 5 cm (on paperback books or video cassette boxes). Gradually increase the height over a period of 3 weeks. At the same time, let your shoulders relax backwards.

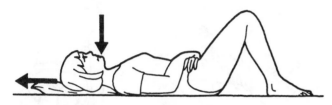

Fig. 2.106 An exercise to stretch the back of your neck and strengthen the front of your neck: Lie down on one pillow. Tuck in your chin, at the same time pushing your neck down and 'lengthening' it.

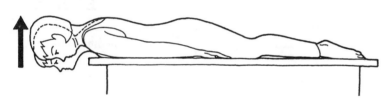

Fig. 2.107 A more advanced postural exercise for younger people: Tuck in your chin as you lift up your head.

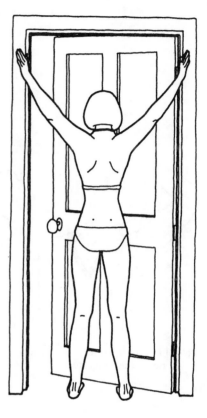

Fig. 2.108 A stretch for round shoulders: Push your chest forwards and hold the stretch for 12 seconds.

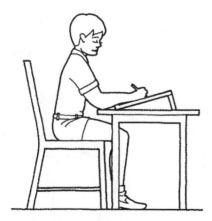

Fig. 2.109 Good writing posture: Bend forwards at the *hips*, not the back. If necessary, use a backrest (*see* Fig. 2.73).

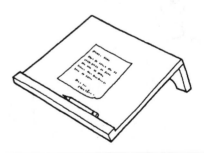

Fig. 2.110 Detail of writing slope.

- **Exercises for VDU (visual display unit) users** (*see* also Fig. 2.117):
  The exercises shown in Figs 2.111–2.116 should be done regularly during the day to prevent neck and backache and headaches.

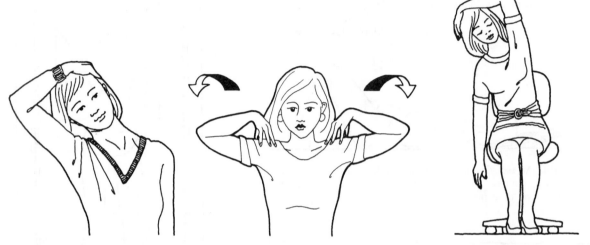

Fig. 2.111 Stretch one side of your neck, then the other.

Fig. 2.112 Circle your elbows backwards.

Fig. 2.113 Stretch one side of your back, then the other.

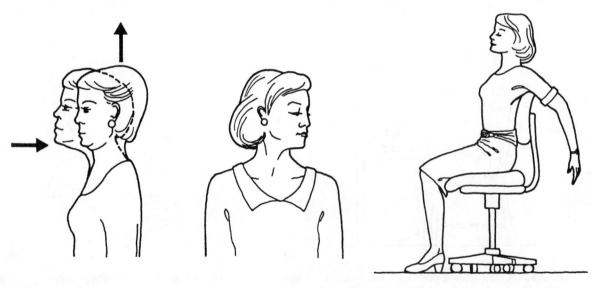

Fig. 2.114 Tuck in your chin, and lengthen the back of your neck.

Fig. 2.115 Tuck in your chin, then turn your head from side to side.

Fig. 2.116 Stretch backwards over the edge of your backrest.

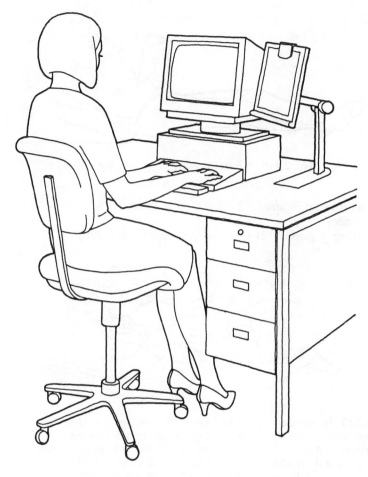

Fig. 2.117 Correct posture at a VDU.

- **Posture in bed**: Figures 2.118 and 2.119 show poor and improved positions for reading in bed. *See* also 'Neck comfort' on pp. 54–56.

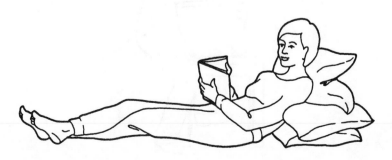

Fig. 2.118 Poor posture when reading in bed.

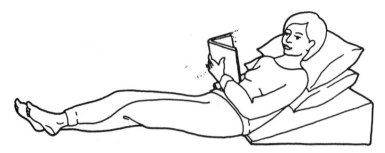

Fig. 2.119 A better posture when reading in bed.

- **Swimming**: Figure 2.120 shows how breaststroke can put a strain on the neck.
- **Lifting**: Figure 2.121 gives advice regarding lifting.

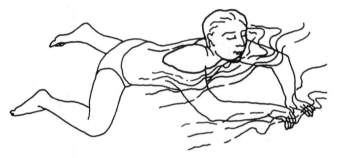

Fig. 2.120 Breaststroke – poor technique: Breaststroke done like this puts a strain on the neck. At the end of swimming a length, move your neck in the opposite direction (*see* Fig. 2.104). It is worth taking lessons to learn a better technique involving a downward pull (rather than an outward pull) of the arms into the water and keeping your head down in the water.

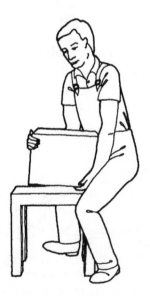

Fig. 2.121 Tuck in your chin every time you lift.

3
Posture

In this chapter, we will look at ways of maintaining the natural curves in our spine when lying down, sitting and standing and when we lift.

We all know how aesthetically pleasing it is to see someone with good posture, and you will have realized how your own posture can change depending on whether or not you have backache, or even depending on the mood you are in. There are very few people who have perfect alignment, but the aim should be to get as close to it as you possibly can, not just because you will look better – and younger – if you achieve this, but also because the spine works better when it is not distorted. Good posture does not mean a return to the rigid postures of the Victorian age: it should be quite relaxed, with the spinal curves in a natural, 'neutral' position. But it does require some effort to substitute good posture for the old habitual one which, after all, has taken you some years to acquire!

Whatever age you are, it will help to work at your posture at some stage in your recovery. When you see older people with bent postures, remember that this is usually the end result of years of not bothering about posture. At best, posture correction will speed up your recovery; at worst it will prevent your present posture from getting worse.

Lying down

Nearly a third of our lives is spent in bed, so the surface we lie on has to be right. If you get back or leg pain in bed or on rising in the morning, it could be due to:

- your bed;
- the particular position you lie in;
- moving from one position to another;
- wearing incorrect footwear on the previous day (see p. 62);
- a delayed reaction to what you have been doing during the day.

One position which often aggravates neck or back pain is sleeping on your tummy. This position places your spinal joints in an extreme position and is not recommended as a sleeping position (Fig. 3.1).

Your bed

The word 'orthopaedic' has become meaningless with regard to beds, and it all too often implies that the mattress is *too hard*. As people get older and their backs become stiffer, many find a too-hard bed uncomfortable. If this applies to you, put a duvet, sleeping bag or a 5 cm sheet of foam rubber on top of the mattress to make the bed more comfortable (Fig. 3.2).

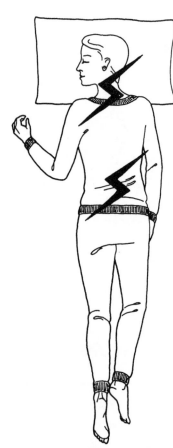

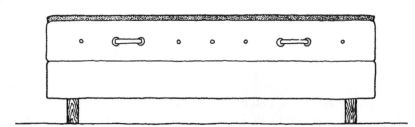

Fig. 3.2 How to make your bed softer. Place a 5 cm sheet of foam rubber or a duvet over the mattress.

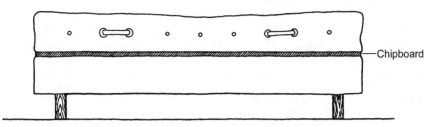

Fig. 3.3 How to make your bed firmer. Place 1½ cm chipboard between base and mattress.

Fig. 3.1 A bad sleeping position: the joints in the back and neck are in an extreme position.

If you are in *acute pain* and every time you move in bed it makes it worse, a firm bed will be more comfortable than one that sags in the middle. But even if your bed is not firm, this is not the right time to invest in a new one. Instead get someone to put 1½ cm chipboard under your mattress (Fig. 3.3), or sleep on a mattress on the floor (provided you can get up and down from it). Don't be tempted to sleep on the floor itself as you would be unable to relax your muscles.

Guidelines on choosing a new bed

Look for a bed that will maintain the natural curves of your spine. Beds don't last for ever – usually the mattress wears out before the base. To prolong the life of your mattress, it should be turned every 6 months. Before going to the expense of buying a new bed, make sure you know the degree of firmness your back likes. Experiment by, for example, sleeping in the spare bed first. If both the base and the mattress of your bed are worn out, the following tips will help you in choosing a new bed:

- The base should be firm, for example wooden slats.
- A medium-firm mattress with individual pocket springs often suits people with stiff spines or people who have a curvature in the spine ('scoliosis').

- People with hypermobility (excessive movement) in their spines often prefer a very firm mattress such as one made from thick foam-rubber.
- Older people are often better with a softer, more yielding mattress.
- With respect to double beds, if there is a big difference in weight between you and your partner, or if each of you prefers a different type of mattress, a good solution is two single beds pushed close together with mattresses to suit each of you.

Pain relief positions

If your back pain is made worse by *bending*, see which of the positions shown in Figs 3.4–3.9 helps you.

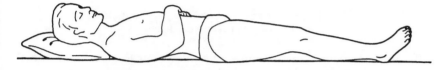

Fig. 3.4 Low back slightly arched.

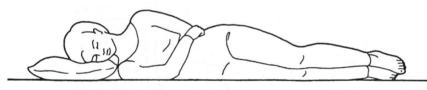

Fig. 3.5 Low back in a 'neutral' position with side lying.

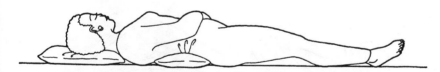

Fig. 3.6 Low back arched more: As well as a pillow under your low back, you may also need to add a second pillow under your head.

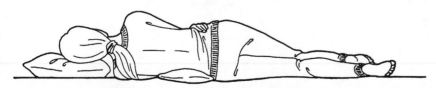

Fig. 3.7 To prevent side-bending: Put a pillow or rolled up towel in your waist.

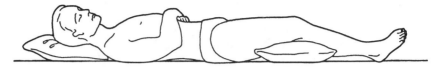

Fig. 3.8 Low back in a 'neutral' position.

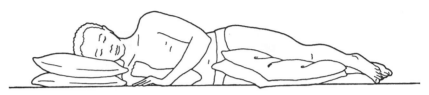

Fig. 3.9 To prevent twisting your low back: Put one or
two pillows between your knees.

If your back pain is made worse by *arching* your low back, try one of
the positions shown in Figs 3.10–3.12.

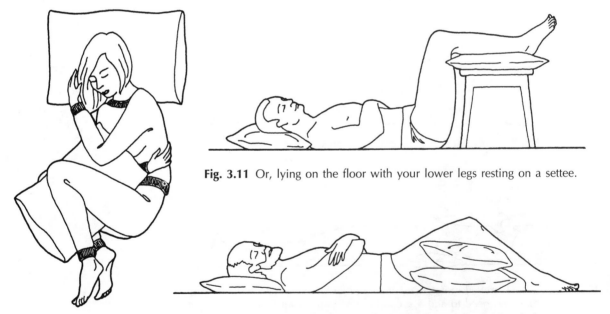

Fig. 3.11 Or, lying on the floor with your lower legs resting on a settee.

Fig. 3.10 'Fetal' position.

Fig. 3.12 A pillow under the knees flattens the back a little.

The correct way to get in and out of bed

Figures 3.13–3.15 illustrate the correct way to get in and out of bed. Some people find the method shown in Fig. 3.16 easier.

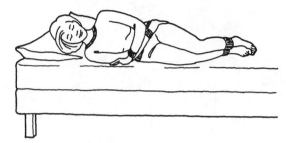

Fig. 3.13 Bend up your hips and knees, then roll on to your side all in one piece.

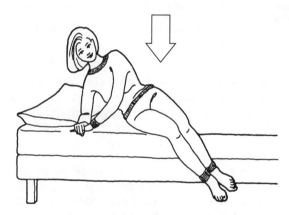

Fig. 3.14 Lift your legs over the side of the bed and push with your hands into the sitting position.

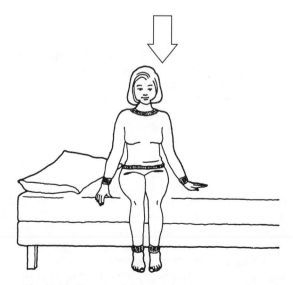

Fig. 3.15 Reverse the procedure for getting into bed.

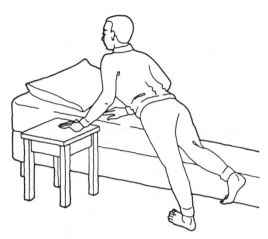

Fig. 3.16 First turn over on to your tummy and then, keeping your back straight, push with your arms as you lower your legs on to the floor.

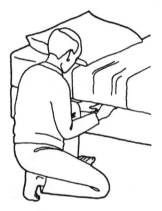

Fig. 3.17 Kneel down and tighten your tummy muscles to protect your back.

Bedmaking

If your back is extra-sensitive when you get up, leave the bedmaking until later in the day. A duvet and fitted sheets make light work of bed-making. Figure 3.17 shows correct posture for bedmaking.

Hotel beds

Be fussy about the bed you sleep in when away on business or on holiday. A saggy bed can set off a bout of back pain, especially after you have been travelling for miles. Hoteliers are often happy to provide a board to go under the mattress, if asked in advance.

Neck comfort

Sleeping on your tummy can *cause* joint problems in the neck because it squashes the joints on one side, while those on the other side are over-stretched. This sleeping position can be responsible for headaches, dizzi-ness, numbness ('deadness') or pins and needles in your arms. If you habitually sleep in this position, you must make every effort to stop or your neck pain may get worse and worse. Simply being determined not to sleep on your tummy works over a period of time – don't give up!

Pillows

Feather pillows flatten down over the years as the feathers lose their curl. To test if a feather pillow has any life in it, punch it in the middle to see if it springs back into shape: if it doesn't, the pillow will have lost a lot of its support. A down pillow is ideal for tucking into the neck for sup-port but they are expensive. Foam chips often aggravate an acutely painful neck by causing too much movement.

Specially contoured pillows are available which support the neck in its natural ('neutral') position (Fig. 3.18) – it is more sensible to try one out

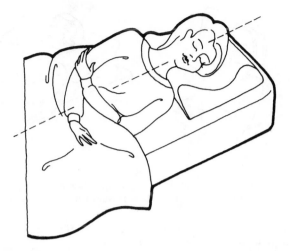

Fig. 3.18 Neck 'in line' using a specially contoured pillow.

first before purchasing it. Some temporary measures are also useful for supporting your neck (Figs 3.19, 3.20).

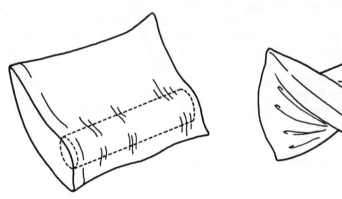

Fig. 3.19 Foam roll inside pillow case.

Fig. 3.20 A 'butterfly' pillow: first twist the pillow, then put it inside your pillowcase.

If you sleep on your side, the width of your shoulders should determine how many pillows you need. If you have broad shoulders you may need two to keep your neck 'in line' (Fig. 3.21). Older people with bent, fixed spines may need two or three pillows if they sleep on their backs to accommodate the shape of the spine. Having too few pillows would be uncomfortable for them.

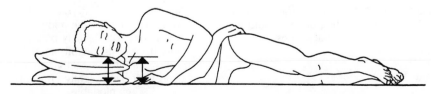

Fig. 3.21 You may need two pillows if you have broad shoulders.

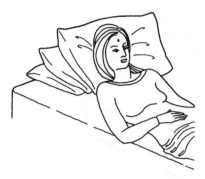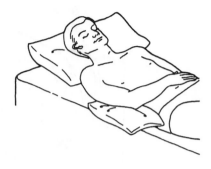

Fig. 3.22 Comfortable position to relieve 'nerve' pain in the arm.

Fig. 3.23 Another pain relieving position for 'nerve' pain in the arm.

People who have 'nerve' pain in the arm may find that one of the positions shown in Figs 3.22 and 3.23 relieve it.

Sitting

The amount of pressure that goes through your back when you sit is surprisingly high and this is why sitting for long periods bothers most people with back pain. This pressure is reduced if the low back is well supported, and increased if you sit in soft, low chairs or settees. It is impossible to sit properly in a chair that is not right for you, so if you are going to sit for any length of time, do be choosy about which chair you sit in if you have the choice. This is particularly important if you have to sit all day at a meeting or if you use a VDU, and also when you sit down in the evening to relax.

How to find a comfortable sitting position

Figures 3.24–3.26 illustrate how to find a comfortable sitting position.

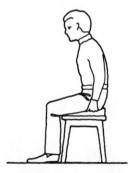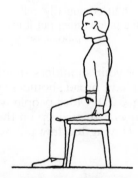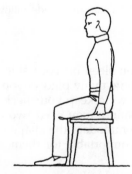

Fig. 3.24 On a firm, level surface (or sitting on a posture wedge as shown), sit on your hands with your palms facing upwards. Feel the bones in the middle of each buttock – your 'sitting bones'. Now slouch – notice that these bones move forwards.

Fig. 3.25 Next, overarch your back – your sitting bones should move backwards.

Fig. 3.26 Stop when you feel that you are sitting on the middle of these bones. This usually puts your low back in its natural 'neutral' position, but if it is painful, arch or bend your back slightly until it is comfortable.

- Now feel the weight of your trunk going *down* through your sitting bones, without letting your back collapse.
- Lift up your rib cage at the front – don't overarch your back while you do this.
- Gently relax your shoulders down and backwards.
- Finally, bring your head back 'in line' with your trunk, tucking in your chin a little. Feel the back of your neck lengthening as if your head is being lifted up from the back of your ears.

The correct posture may feel a little strange at first but if you practise this regime for two 10-minute sessions a day it will soon become second nature.

Working with VDUs

Figure 3.27 shows a well designed work-station.

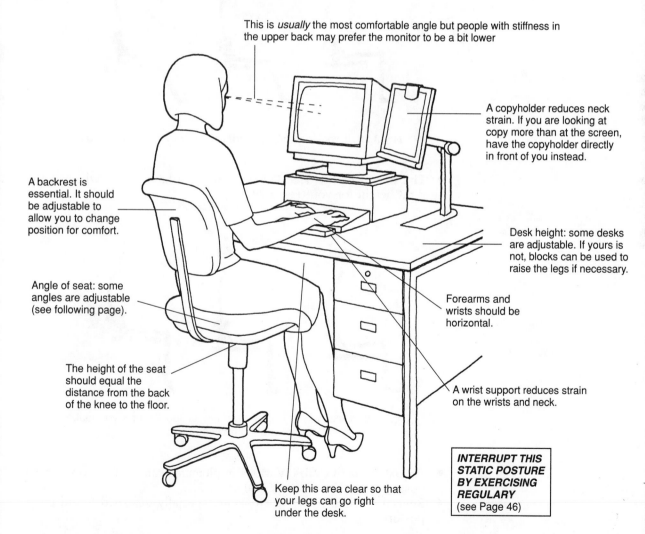

This is *usually* the most comfortable angle but people with stiffness in the upper back may prefer the monitor to be a bit lower

A copyholder reduces neck strain. If you are looking at copy more than at the screen, have the copyholder directly in front of you instead.

A backrest is essential. It should be adjustable to allow you to change position for comfort.

Desk height: some desks are adjustable. If yours is not, blocks can be used to raise the legs if necessary.

Angle of seat: some angles are adjustable (see following page).

Forearms and wrists should be horizontal.

The height of the seat should equal the distance from the back of the knee to the floor.

A wrist support reduces strain on the wrists and neck.

Keep this area clear so that your legs can go right under the desk.

INTERRUPT THIS STATIC POSTURE BY EXERCISING REGULARLY (see Page 46)

Fig. 3.27 A well designed work-station. It is important to interrupt this static posture by exercising regularly (*see* p. 46).

Your chair

- **Moving in your chair**: Use your feet to manoeuvre your swivel chair to avoid twisting your back.
- **Armrests** are useful for support: they should go *under* your desk, otherwise you will be too far away from it.
- **Footrests** are necessary if your feet do not reach floor level; they also tend to help people who are more comfortable with a *flat* back. Those who prefer to sit with an *arched* back may find that a footrest is unnecessary.
- **The angle of the seat**: Vary this if it is adjustable (Fig. 3.28).

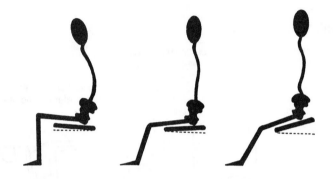

Fig. 3.28 If your seat angle is adjustable, vary it during the day.

- **The height of the seat**: It is important to have a seat which is the right height for you (Fig. 3.29).

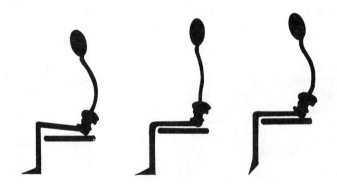

Fig. 3.29 A seat which is either too low or too high for you makes your spine bend.

- **Adjustments to chairs**: Various implements can be used to improve posture when sitting (Figs 3.30 and 3.31).
- **Special seating**: Kneeling stools are specially designed to aid good posture (Fig. 3.32).

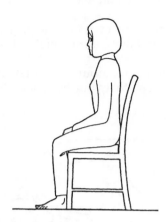

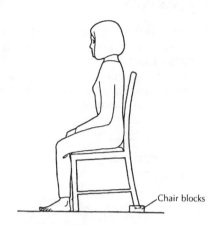

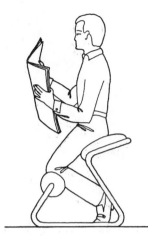

Fig. 3.30 A posture wedge helps to straighten the back.

Fig. 3.31 Chair blocks under the back legs help to straighten the back.

Fig. 3.32 The kneeling stool also helps you to keep a straight back. Although it reduces disc pressure, it should only be used for short periods. A backrest is essential if you sit for longer periods.

Writing

Figures 3.33 and 3.34 show good and bad positions for writing.

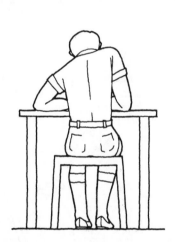

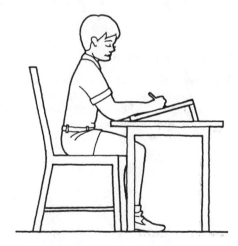

Fig. 3.33 Awkward position when writing.

Fig. 3.34 The use of a writing slope helps to prevent the neck and back bending.

Driving

Figures 3.35 and 3.36 show bad and good driving posture. There are other points of advice/information worth noting:

- Pressing the clutch increases disc pressure.
- An automatic car is better for chronic *left-sided* back pain.
- Power-assisted steering is better for people with chronic neck or back problems.

- Check that your pedals are not offset: this would make you twist your back.
- The headrest should be on a level with your eyes for safety.
- Make sure you sit squarely on the seat, taking even weight on your buttocks.
- On long journeys, stop every hour and walk around for a few minutes. Also, vary the rake of the backrest so that your back doesn't get 'set' in one position.

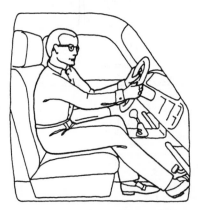

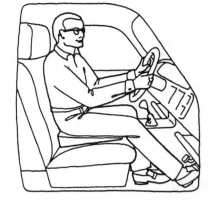

Fig. 3.35 Tense driving posture: a bent back puts high pressure on your discs.

Fig. 3.36 A posture wedge to level the seat or a lumbar support (*see* Fig. 2.45) helps to straighten your back.

Sitting for relaxation

Most settees should be banned! They are usually too deep and too soft, which encourages slouching. A supportive chair is better for you (Figs 3.37 and 3.38). The backrest should slope *backwards* (a vertical backrest does not give sufficient support).

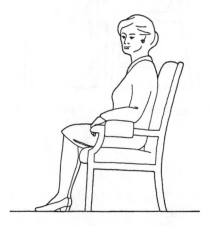

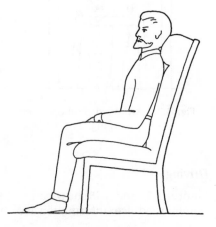

Fig. 3.37 Proper arm support encourages you to make good use of the backrest, and helps you to get up from the chair.

Fig. 3.38 Good neck support – particularly useful if you tend to doze off in your chair.

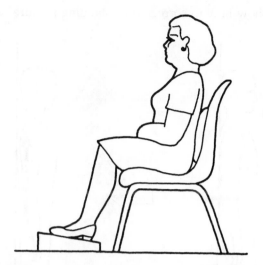

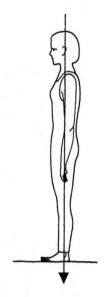

Fig. 3.39 A 'bucket' type of chair can be improved by using a lumbar support and footstool.

Fig. 3.40 Back 'in line' with ideal curves.

Lumbar supports come in all shapes and sizes – there is no 'right' or 'wrong' – choose one that suits your particular back and put it in whichever part of your back feels more comfortable. Figure 3.39 illustrates the use of a lumbar support and footstool.

Standing and walking

Standing still can be uncomfortable for people with back problems. The longer we stand, the more the low back tends to arch, causing backache. Ideally, our spines should be gently curved as in Fig. 3.40. You will see, however, that the shape of people's backs varies a lot. Is yours like any of those in Figs 3.41–3.44?

Different types of backs

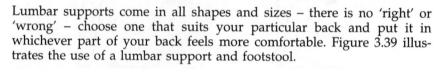

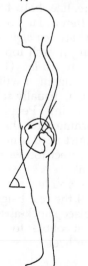

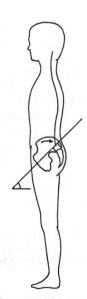

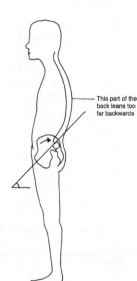

This part of the back leans too far backwards

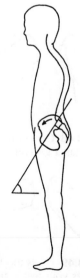

Fig. 3.41 Exaggerated curves.

Fig. 3.42 Flat back.

Fig. 3.43 'Sway' back.

Fig. 3.44 Round back.

Figures 3.45–3.47 show how to correct your standing posture.

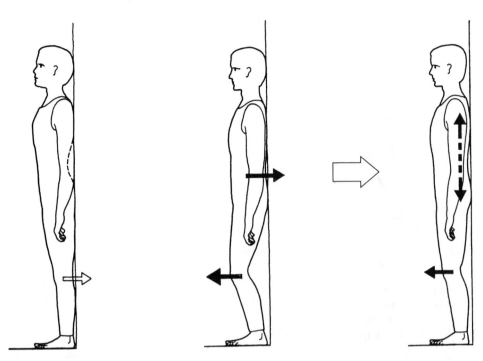

Fig. 3.45 'Military type' posture: This posture is too rigid.

Fig. 3.46 Start with your *feet*. Transfer some weight on to the outside of your feet and on to your heels. Let your knees relax forwards slightly, and gently pull in your tummy muscles.

Fig. 3.47 Correct standing posture: Relax your shoulder blades downwards and inwards, and raise your rib cage at the front. Gently tuck in your chin, lengthening your whole spine.

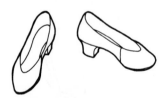

Fig. 3.48 Correct heel height (as a general rule).

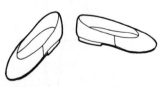

Fig. 3.49 Heels too low: This causes your feet – and legs – to roll in, arching your back.

Footwear

This can cause more problems than most people realize, both for men and women! The *height* of your heels makes a big difference to your back (Figs 3.48–3.50). Most people know that if the heels are *too high* (over 4 cm or 2 inches), this will affect the back by making it arch too much. What is less obvious, however, is that if the heels are *too low* (1 cm or less) this will also have a marked effect on the back – again, it will make it arch too much, eventually causing backache. This is usually felt *after* standing or *after* walking – you may be sitting at the time! People often get pain in bed or on waking on the following morning after they have been wearing incorrect footwear, and think they must need a new bed. Because there is a delayed reaction to wearing incorrect footwear, it is not surprising that most people miss the connection!

A heel may appear to be higher than it actually is – you have to deduct the thickness of the sole from that of the heel to find the real height. An easy way of raising the height of your heels is to place shock-absorbing heel pads inside your shoes (*see* Fig. 3.60), or to ask a cobbler to stick on one-eighth to a quarter of an inch of rubber on each heel.

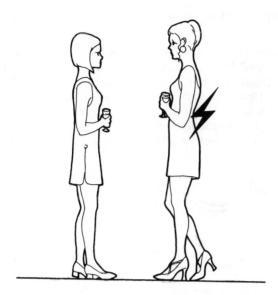

Fig. 3.50 Effect of heel height on back posture.

How your *feet* affect your back

Nowadays we spend a lot of time standing and walking on hard, unyielding surfaces such as pavements. To prevent jolts going up into the back,
our feet should act as shock absorbers. But this can only happen if our
feet function in the right way, and to do this they need to have an **arch**
(instep).

Some people are born with flat feet and they frequently get backache
because of this. Most people's feet have an arch when they are not bear-
ing weight but, when they stand, either one or both feet roll inwards
causing the foot/feet to flatten. This has a 'knock-on effect' on the back:
with every step taken – and it is estimated that we take about 5000 steps
a day – the back is jolted, and small jolts all add up.

Stand in front of a mirror and look at your feet. Do they have an arch
(Fig. 3.51)? Or does one foot (or both) roll inwards, flattening the arch
(Fig. 3.52)? If either one or both feet roll inwards, this makes your foot
– and leg – roll inwards too, throwing the weight too far forwards on to
the balls of your feet. Your low back then has to arch too much to keep
you upright.

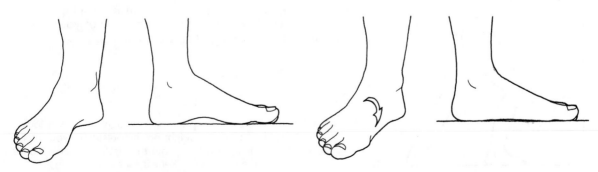

Fig. 3.51 Feet with good arches.   **Fig. 3.52** Flat feet.

Two things will help this situation:

1. Wearing shoes with a suitable heel height (Figs 3.48, 3.53).
2. Wearing **orthotics** (Fig. 3.54) in your shoes. These are insoles which can be prescribed by a physiotherapist specializing in orthotics (*see* p. 96 for address) or a podiatrist, and they can be very beneficial in correcting foot posture and preventing your back being jarred with every step you take. Although temporary, 'off the peg' orthotics are available, the custom-made ones which are fabricated using a cast of your feet are more effective and more comfortable to wear.

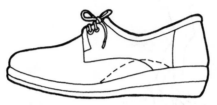

Fig. 3.53 A good shoe (the heel need not necessarily be wedge-shaped).

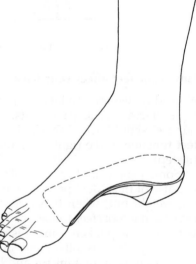

Fig. 3.54 An orthotic device: This is different from just an arch support.

Keeping your ankles supple will help prevent your feet rolling in. Figure 3.55 shows an ankle stretch to achieve this. If only one of your feet rolls in, this has the effect of 'shortening' that leg (*see* p. 65).

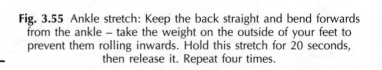

Fig. 3.55 Ankle stretch: Keep the back straight and bend forwards from the ankle – take the weight on the outside of your feet to prevent them rolling inwards. Hold this stretch for 20 seconds, then release it. Repeat four times.

Short leg

It is probably more common than not to have legs of unequal length. We rarely notice this ourselves until someone points it out to us. If, say, the right leg is shorter than the left, the spine has to compensate for this by curving (Fig. 3.56). People tend to stand with more weight on the short leg side (Fig. 3.57).

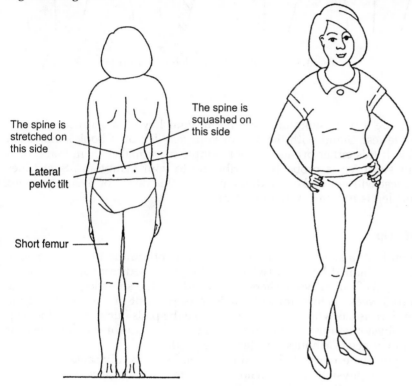

The spine is stretched on this side

The spine is squashed on this side

Lateral pelvic tilt

Short femur

Fig. 3.56 A short left leg.

Fig. 3.57 Standing posture with short left leg.

To check if your legs are of even length

- Stand in front of a long mirror with your feet together.
- Put your hands on your hip bones and see if they are level (*see* Fig. 3.58). If they aren't, look at your knees – are they level?
- If your knees are level but your hip bones are not, you may have a shorter thigh bone (as in Fig. 3.58).
- If one knee and hip on the same side are both lower, look at your ankle bones. Is one ankle bone lower than the other? If it is, then this is probably due to the foot rolling in on that side, shortening that leg.

Symptoms

These usually come on gradually. You may feel stiffness, an ache or pain, either on the side of the short leg or the long leg, or in the midline (Fig. 3.59). The symptoms usually come on while walking or running. Sometimes they are felt afterwards – either when sitting, or in bed at night, or even the following morning.

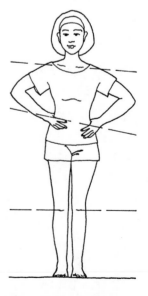

Fig. 3.58 Checking for a short leg.

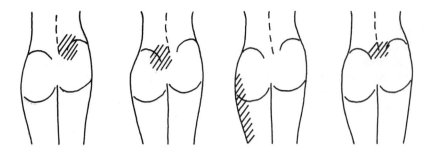

Fig. 3.59 Site of symptoms due to a short leg.

To see if your symptoms are due to your having a short leg, try this simple test. Stand with the foot of your *long* leg on a book about 1 cm thick. If this either brings on your symptoms or makes them *worse*, then your short leg is probably contributing to your symptoms. Sometimes this test will not make any difference, but this does not mean that your short leg is not part of the problem.

Self-help

If you have a short leg and you think it *is* contributing to your problem, put a cushioned heel pad (which can be purchased from sports shops – *see* Fig. 3.60) in all your shoes on the side of the short leg. It may take up to 3 weeks before any noticeable improvement in pain occurs. If the pain *increases* or you feel a new pain, take the pads out and seek the help of a physiotherapist. The pain may either be due to some other cause, or you may need orthotics (insoles) – *see* p. 64.

If you have marked shortening of one leg, it is advisable for you to consult a physiotherapist, who will be able to advise you concerning appropriate adjustments to your footwear.

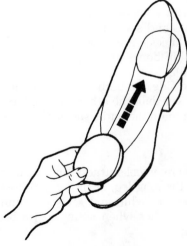

Fig. 3.60 Use of a cushioned heel pad: This can be used for (a) raising the shoe of a short leg or (b) preventing jarring (if legs are of even length, place a pad in *both* shoes).

Lifting

Pressure on your back

Lifting increases the pressure on the discs in your back, even if it is done carefully. When ligaments or discs have been damaged or if the back is acutely painful, lifting in the early stages of healing can cause further damage and so should be avoided during this time. If one of your discs has been damaged, your back will be particularly over-sensitive during the first few hours after rising in the morning, so avoid lifting during this risky period. Also, after sitting for a long time, especially after driving, don't lift immediately afterwards.

During the process of healing, the back will gradually be able to cope with more pressure. Nevertheless, everyone should discover how much he/she is capable of lifting *safely*. Pain should be the main guide – but remember that sometimes there is a delayed reaction: it may not be until the following morning that you feel the effect of lifting.

Repetitive lifting causes fluid to be squeezed from your discs, flattening them slightly and making the facet joints rub together (Fig. 3.61). Wearing a corset or weight-lifter's belt can help prevent this (Fig. 3.62). Giving your back a 20 minute rest periodically reduces the pressure and allows your discs to reinflate, taking the stress off your facet joints (Fig. 3.63). Indeed, it would do everyone's back a great deal of good if they could have a siesta every day!

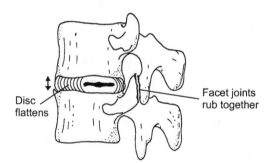

Disc flattens

Facet joints rub together

Fig. 3.61 Effect of repetitive lifting.

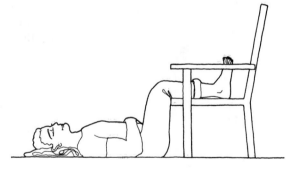

Fig. 3.63 The ideal position to reinflate your discs.

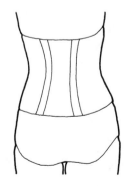

Fig. 3.62 A corset or weight-lifter's belt can reduce the pressure on your back when you lift, but don't become dependent on one.

Leverage

NEVER lift with outstretched arms: this makes your back muscles work much harder because of increased leverage, which can increase disc pressure so much that it damages your discs. The illustrations in Fig. 3.64 show how much the back muscles work with the arms in different positions.

> It is very important to *get close to what you are lifting*.

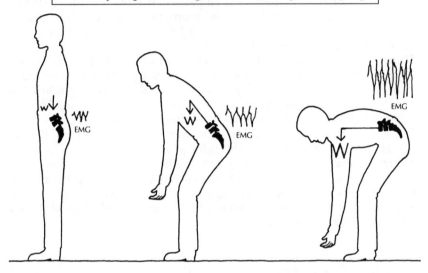

Fig. 3.64 A load requires increased back muscle activity (as indicated by the EMG traces) when it is held further in front of the body.

Preparing to lift

In order to lift properly, you need strong knees. Semi-squats are a good way of strengthening them (Fig. 3.65) and then, every time you lift correctly, you will keep them strong.

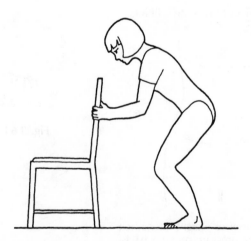

Fig. 3.65 Semi-squats: Slowly lower yourself into this position (not into a *full* squat), then straighten up again.

General guidelines

• If possible use a hoist or other mechanical device.

• Cluttered areas cause you to *lean and lift* which is very bad for your back.

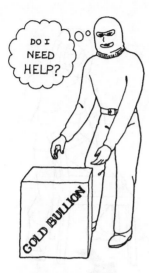

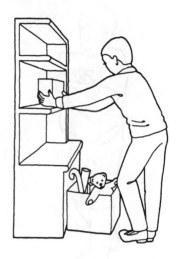

PLAN THE LIFT

KEEP THE AREA TIDY

- Don't wear your best clothes to move dirty objects!
- Wear clothes that are loose enough so that you can move freely, but tight enough to avoid catching.
- Wear gloves, if necessary, to protect your hands.

- Heavy loads should NOT be lifted repetitively from *floor level* – they should be placed between *knee and shoulder*.

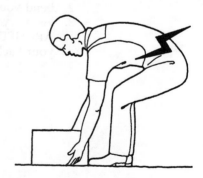

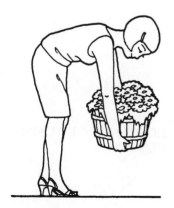

BE CAREFUL WHEN LIFTING LOADS FROM THE FLOOR

WEAR SUITABLE CLOTHING!

- The closer you are to the load, the lower the disc pressure.

- If possible, get the load between your knees.
- Get a good grip.
- Face the direction in which you intend to move.

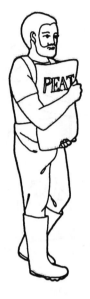

GET CLOSE TO THE LOAD!

MOVE YOUR FEET: DON'T TWIST YOUR BACK!

- When you lift:
  1. tuck in your chin;
  2. bend your knees a little;
  3. keep your back STRAIGHT, not ARCHED (this does *not* mean keeping your back vertical).

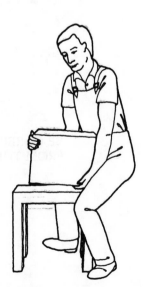

TIGHTEN YOUR TUMMY MUSCLES

Carrying

Carrying has a similar effect on the back to lifting, except that the effect on the discs is more gradual. Thus, the sensible way to shop is to use a trolley (Fig. 3.66).

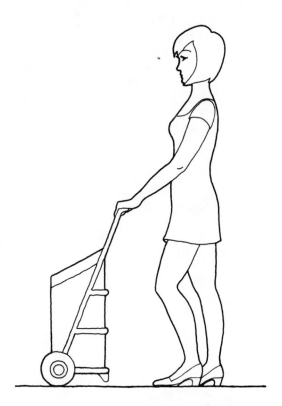

Fig. 3.66 A shopping trolley: These are now becoming much more 'trendy' and reduce back and neck strain considerably.

4
First aid for your back

What to do if your back seizes up

Hopefully, the advice in the preceding pages will prevent, or at least reduce the likelihood of, you having a sudden seizure of back pain. But what should you do if this does happen and you get stuck in one position? Indeed, this may be the reason you bought this book: to find out the answer to this question.

Hard though it may be, try not to panic – this simply makes things much worse. Your instinct will be to hold on to something for support – so do that – be it a chair, table, even your legs. Then keep perfectly still. The initial sharp pain will ease a little, and when it does, *slowly* try to straighten up by 'walking' your hands up your legs. Don't force any movement. The best thing to do next is to lie down on a firm, supportive surface – a bed, if you can – preferably *not* the floor unless there's no alternative: getting up from the floor can be extremely difficult when you're in pain. Also, the floor is too hard for comfort. Lie in whatever position is comfortable for you. You do not necessarily have to lie flat on your back, unless this position relieves the pain. Choose one of the resting positions shown on pp. 51–52 but make adjustments to suit yourself if you need to. It is usually best *not* to rest in a chair because sitting puts high pressure on the back, so even if it feels comfortable to begin with, you may be causing further damage.

A home-made ice-pack, such as a bag of frozen peas, applied over the painful area for 10 minutes every few hours, often gives relief from pain.

The amount of rest you need in the early stages depends on how much damage has been done to your back. Let pain be your guide: it is nature's way of warning you that if you continue to perform a particular movement or activity, further damage will occur. Don't be heroic. If it is painful to stand or sit, then lie down. Try to 'listen' to your back and give it what it needs – then it will recover more quickly. It is surprising how anxiety about the situation can make the pain a lot worse: if you tense your muscles, they will cause more pressure on the painful area, so try to relax. The relaxation exercise on p. 92 is useful: you can do it in any position that is comfortable. Comfort yourself with the thought that the majority of back pain clears up within 3 days.

When to stay on bedrest

Relatively few people need to stay on bedrest for longer than 3 days, but there is one important exception and that is when a disc has been badly damaged (*see* pp. 17–28). The back or leg pain (sciatica) is severe and may be constant in the first few days. The slightest movement hurts. Bedrest may then be necessary for between a few days and 3 weeks, depending on how quickly the pain subsides. It is not uncommon for the pain to increase during the first 24 hours, despite bedrest, because injury causes swelling inside the back and this irritates sensitive nerves. Usually the intensity of pain will then start to decrease.

When to call your family doctor

In the following circumstances, you should ask your doctor to visit you at home:

- If the pain is intolerable.
- If the pain starts to spread from your back into one or both legs.
- If you have 'deadness' or 'numbness' in one or both legs.
- If you are unable to urinate (pass water).
- If your foot or leg feels weak.

Signs of recovery

Be patient. Don't expect the pain to disappear suddenly; it is usually a gradual process. If one or more of the following happen, this indicates that recovery is starting:

- The pain will be less intense.
- The area of pain will lessen.
- The pain will be felt closer to the back rather than, for example, in the leg or buttock.
- It will be easier to move and you will be able to stand and walk for increasingly longer periods before the pain comes on.

During the recovery period, make sure that you have plenty of magazines, books etc. to keep you occupied – but don't sit up in bed to read them! At first, only get up when you need to go to the toilet. A man can use a bottle to urinate, if necessary, but it is not so easy for a woman! *See* Figs 3.13–3.16 for the correct way to get in and out of bed. If walking is painful, use crutches or sticks (or even a broom!) to help you to get to the toilet. It may be less traumatic for you to crawl rather than walk. You will need help during this period, so don't be too proud to ask a friend or relative to do chores such as shopping, food preparation etc. for you.

While on bedrest, eat easily digestible food so that you do not have to strain when you go to the toilet. In the early stages, don't be tempted to lie in a hot bath: this would allow the back to bend too much and you may get stuck there.

Correct breathing

When you are lying down, you may tend to 'shallow breathe' all the time because your lungs don't have to fully expand when you are resting. However, this means that less oxygen is taken in. Your body needs a good supply of oxygen to help it to heal and for normal body functions, so it is important for you to practise deep breathing. To do this:

- Let your shoulders relax.
- Put one hand on the front of your waist and, as you breathe in, let the air come right down to your waist so that you expand here, like a balloon (Fig. 4.1). Breathe in to a count of four.
- Now slowly and effortlessly breathe out to a count of six: you should now feel your hand coming in towards your body.

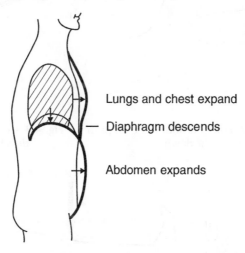

Lungs and chest expand

Diaphragm descends

Abdomen expands

Fig. 4.1 The correct way to breathe. (Reprinted from *Your health at the VDU: a practical guide to reducing physical stress at the workplace*, a booklet by Sheila Marks and Jean Oliver, published in 1966 by Health Monitoring Unit Ltd. Ilustration by Martin Sandhill.)

Do this for about a minute, every hour. This is the correct way to breathe anyway and it is very relaxing, so if you are feeling tense, check to see that you are using your lungs correctly in this manner.

Self-help is different depending on what you have done to your back. Read pp. 9–40 and follow the appropriate advice and exercises. If you are in any doubt whatsoever about what to do, contact a chartered physiotherapist.

Exercises to do when on bedrest

In addition to the exercises which are given under the appropriate syndrome, it is important to do gentle exercises for the rest of your body to keep it supple and to keep some tone in your muscles. It has been shown that this makes a big difference to the rate of recovery. Figures 4.2–4.7 show suitable exercises to do on bedrest. Try to do ten of each of these exercises (on both sides of the body) every hour during the day. These exercises must *not* be painful; if any of them does cause pain, miss it out.

When to return to everyday activities

It is not sensible to go straight from bedrest to doing normal, everyday activities. Your muscles will have weakened even if you have done some gentle exercises while on bedrest. As the pain subsides, you can start

Exercises to do when on bedrest

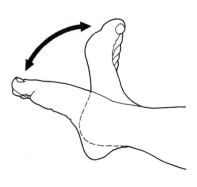

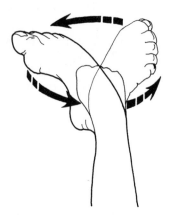

Fig. 4.2 Pull your foot up, then push it down.

Fig. 4.3 Circle your foot round in one direction, then the other.

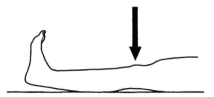

Fig. 4.4 Brace your knee back and hold for 10 seconds, then relax.

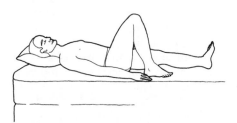

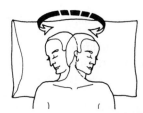

Fig. 4.5 Gently bend up one knee, then straighten your leg again, keeping your heel down.

Fig. 4.6 Gently roll your head to one side, then the other.

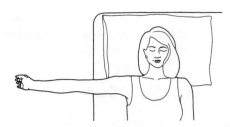

Fig. 4.7 Straighten out one arm to the side, bending the wrist back, then bend up again.

controlled activity. This means doing an activity for a short period only and then resting *before* the pain comes on. If you don't get a delayed, painful reaction you may be safe to attempt the activity for slightly longer. In this way, the strength of your muscles will be built up gradually. Being able to sit comfortably is usually a problem to start with. You will find that sitting on a dining chair is more comfortable than on a lower, soft chair. A posture wedge and/or backrest (see p. 23) often make sitting more comfortable. Avoid sofas: you can't help but slouch in them.

Driving

The car seat may need similar adjustments (see above), as these seats usually slope backwards. If you are unsure as to whether it is safe for you to drive, then be a passenger first, for a short journey (e.g. 5–10 minutes), and see how you fare. Remember that driving itself will put even higher pressure on your back because of depressing the clutch pedal in particular.

Everyday activities

Analyse what movements are involved in normal, everyday activities and it will give you an idea of whether you are ready to attempt them. Hoovering, for instance, involves lifting the hoover out – usually from awkward corners (probably involving twisting or reaching), and then pushing. An upright hoover is usually easier on the back than one which causes you to bend a lot. Walk close to the hoover to avoid stretching out. Ironing involves standing and leaning forwards slightly, plus a little bit of twisting. Have the ironing board as high as possible, but don't be tempted to do all of the ironing at once!

Sexual intercourse

This rather depends, too, on how understanding your partner is. If your back prefers to be straight rather than bent forwards, you will be better on top of your partner. If you are more comfortable with your back flat or bent you will be better underneath with your knees bent and maybe a pillow under your buttocks, or even lying on your side. Once the acute pain has subsided, it is not necessary to abstain: just use a little ingenuity!

5

Pregnancy and after childbirth

From the third month of pregnancy onwards, hormonal changes occur which affect all the ligaments in the body, making them looser. The spinal ligaments are no exception – indeed, because of the increasing weight carried in front, they are under the most stress. To allow for the expansion of the growing fetus, the ligaments of the pelvis also become looser and do not return to their normal length until up to 6 months after childbirth. Those connecting the two parts of the pelvis together (the sacrum and the ilium) – the sacroiliac ligaments – are the ones that are most frequently strained in pregnancy. However, pain felt in the area of the sacroiliac joint can also come from the spine itself (*see* pp. 18, 25 and 30).

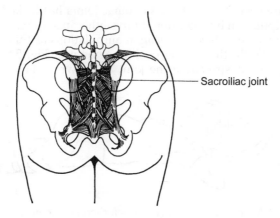

Sacroiliac joint

Fig. 5.1 The sacroiliac joints.

The sacroiliac joints

The sacroiliac joints (Fig. 5.1) have uneven joint surfaces which fit together a bit like your knuckles (Fig. 5.2). Normally very little movement occurs in these joints. However, in the vulnerable period during pregnancy and up to 6 months afterwards when the joints' ligaments are looser, this sometimes enables the joint surfaces to move on each other so that they get stuck in a different position (Fig. 5.3). Women who are naturally hypermobile (turn to p. 12 to see if you are) are more prone to this type of problem, as well as those who are having their second pregnancy or who are expecting twins.

Most commonly, uneven and twisting stresses tend to strain the sacroiliac ligaments.

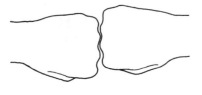

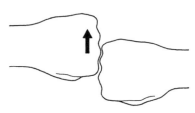

Fig. 5.2 The sacroiliac joint surfaces normally fit together like this.

Fig. 5.3 When the ligaments are loose, the surfaces can move like this and lock the sacroiliac joint in a different position.

Sacroiliac joint problems

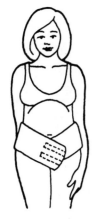

Fig. 5.4 Use of pelvic binder for sacroiliac problems.

If a ligament strain does occur it can be quite incapacitating, being painful on twisting movements such as turning over in bed or simply when taking weight through the leg on the affected side. The ligament may simply be strained, or the joint may be stuck (called a 'locked' joint) as previously described. If it is simply strained, taking it easy for a few days and wearing a pelvic binder (Fig. 5.4) or trochanteric belt for support will help.

However, if one of the sacroiliac joints has locked, it may need gentle manipulation by a chartered physiotherapist to restore correct alignment. It is unwise to have *too many* manipulations as this can make your joints unstable. Resting in the position shown in Fig. 5.5 may help to unlock the joint, or stretching the joint as shown in Fig. 5.6. Wearing a pelvic

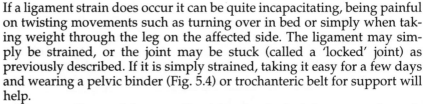

Fig. 5.5 Resting position for the left sacroiliac joint: Lie in this position for 20 minutes.

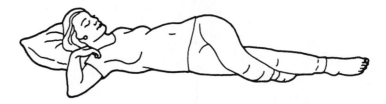

Fig. 5.6 A stretch for the left sacroiliac joint: Gently pull your left knee towards your left shoulder and your left foot towards your right groin.

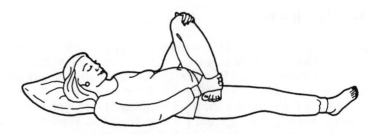

binder *before* manipulation can make the pain worse if the joint is locked in the wrong position, but wearing one *after* manipulation is necessary to maintain the correction.

Prevention of strains

Comfortable resting and sleeping positions

Prevention of strains is all important, especially for those women in the

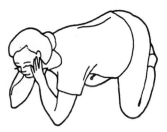

Fig. 5.8

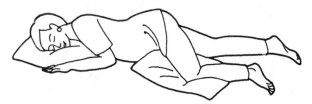

Fig. 5.7

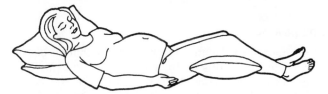

Fig. 5.9

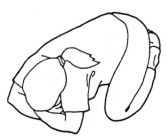

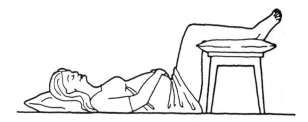

Fig. 5.10

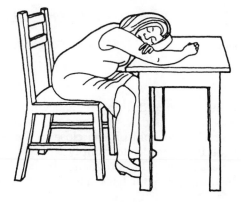

Fig. 5.11

Fig. 5.12

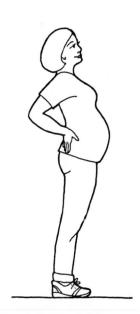

Fig. 5.13 This stretch helps some pregnant women but is not meant to encourage an arched-back posture.

high risk category. To overcome the overwhelming fatigue, the pregnant mother should have a daily rest period, trying one or more of the positions shown in Figs 5.7–5.12. The stretch shown in Fig. 5.13 can also be comfortable and relaxing.

Getting in and out of bed/the car

To protect your sacroiliac joints, press your bent knees together and follow the procedure shown in Figs 3.13–3.15 when getting in and out of bed. Do the same when getting in and out of the car.

Correct standing posture

The shape of the pregnant woman's spine starts to change because the extra weight carried in front pulls on the back. Also, the ligaments holding up the arches of the feet become looser, causing the arches to flatten and making the feet and legs roll in. Both of these factors lead to an increased curve in the low back. Wearing the right type of footwear (*see* pp. 62–64) can help your posture and balance, as well as remembering to hold yourself properly (Figs 5.14, 5.15).

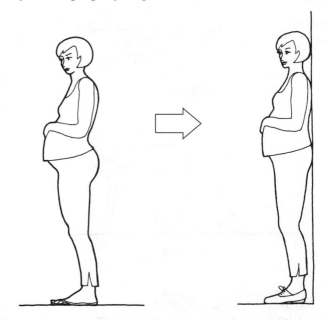

Fig. 5.14 Poor standing posture.   **Fig. 5.15** Correct standing posture.

Lifting

Avoid heavy lifting and carrying during pregnancy if you possibly can – not easy if you also have a toddler. As your size increases, the main rule of safe lifting, which is to hold objects close to the centre of your body (*see* pp. 67–71) becomes harder to comply with.

Strengthen your knees early in the pregnancy by bending from your hips and knees instead of from your back (Fig. 5.16), in preparation for later!

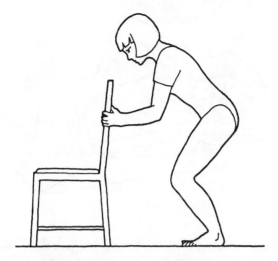

Fig. 5.16 Semi-squats: Slowly lower yourself into this position (not into a full squat), then straighten up again.

Exercise during pregnancy

Moderate exercise is recommended, especially swimming or exercising in a pool – several short sessions per week being more beneficial than one long one. Going for regular, short walks is also a good, natural form of exercise during pregnancy – be sure to wear the right shoes for this.

After the birth

Remember that the ligaments are still loose for up to 6 months and that you still need to take extra care to avoid too much bending and to keep a good posture. Women often tend to sway forwards when standing, even after the baby is born, out of habit, and this can cause long-term problems. Strengthening your over-stretched abdominal muscles has the added bonus of improving your posture, as well as helping your back and making you look good.

Abdominal exercises

While you are on the maternity unit, make a point of seeing the obstetrics physiotherapist so that she can check that you are doing these exercises correctly, as it is easy to cheat without realizing it. If your abdominal muscles are very weak, it may be easier for you to tense them when lying on your side with your knees bent (Fig. 5.17). Don't feel that you have to lie down to do this exercise. As soon as you are able to tense the right muscles, do this exercise when sitting or standing, for example when queuing up in the supermarket! For a progression of this exercise *see* Figs 1.18 and 1.19 on p. 7.

Occasionally the abdominal muscles separate in the midline during pregnancy. If this has happened to you, you should see a chartered physiotherapist who will show you how to support the muscles while you exercise them. She will also measure the gap and monitor improvement.

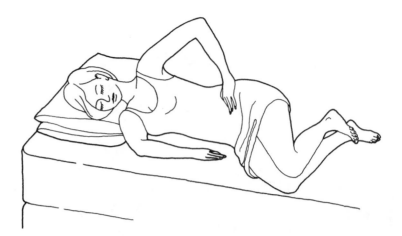

Fig. 5.17 Abdominal exercise: As you breathe *out*, pull in the lower part of your tummy under your tummy button – hold tight for 5 seconds, increasing to 10 seconds as the muscles get stronger. At the same time tighten your pelvic floor muscles between your legs (as if to stop yourself urinating).

Nappy changing

Figures 5.18–5.20 illustrate some good and bad ways to change nappies.

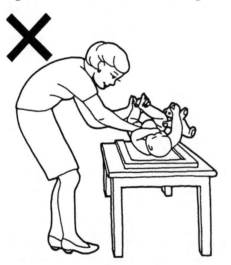

Fig. 5.18 A surface that is too low causes bending of the back.

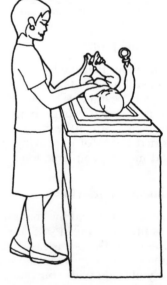

Fig. 5.20 Use a waist-high surface.

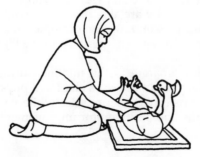

Fig. 5.19 Avoid bending your back, by half-kneeling like this.

Breast feeding

Comfort for the mother is essential during this important activity. Figures 5.21 and 5.22 show two suitable feeding positions.

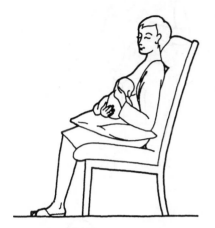

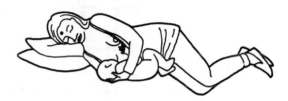

Fig. 5.22 Side-lying is a comfortable position for some mothers.

Fig. 5.21 Support your low back and your baby on a pillow.

Lifting and carrying

Figures 5.23–5.28 illustrate some dos and don'ts with respect to lifting and carrying.

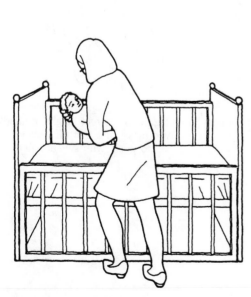

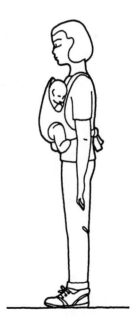

Fig. 5.23 Keep your back as straight as possible. Avoid twisting by standing at a diagonal.

Fig. 5.24 Wear a sling as high as possible, and fix the straps firmly. But remember, the baby gets heavier the more you carry it!

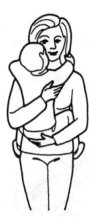

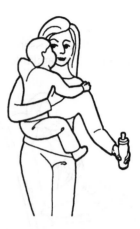

Fig. 5.25 Correct way to carry your child.

Fig. 5.26 Do not carry your child like this!

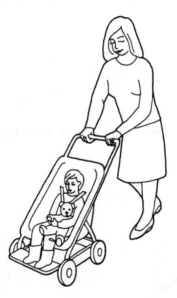

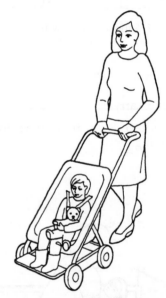

Fig. 5.27 The handles of this buggy are too low.

Fig. 5.28 Correct height of handles. Also make sure that the buggy is easy to push, with swivel wheels.

6
The older back

As we get older, certain changes take place in our spines. The facet joints and ligaments start to stiffen up and our discs become flatter and are then less efficient at absorbing stresses. Flattening of the discs is one of the reasons why we get a bit smaller as we get older; the other being that unless we are very careful we start to stoop.

Fortunately, it is possible to offset some of these changes by exercising our joints to keep them as supple as possible. Exercise should be as natural as possible: regular walking and swimming being the safest, or perhaps joining an over-60's exercise class. The old saying, 'If you don't use it, you lose it' is certainly true as far as our joints are concerned. The good news about our discs is that, provided the discs have not prolapsed, they usually become a lot more stable by the mid-50's, and bouts of severe, incapacitating back seizures are far less common after this age.

Self-help

- Pay attention to your posture (*see* Chapter 3). While it may seem a good idea to keep your low back as straight as possible, some older people find that if they arch their back too much it causes problems. This is why standing still for long periods can cause backache, because it causes the back to arch more – if you can, rest one foot on a block (*see* Fig. 2.70).
- Keep active with *moderate* exercise. It has been proved that regular exercise can help to prevent osteoporosis ('brittle bones'), in combination with healthy eating.

Footwear and feet

It is often necessary to take a fresh look at the type of shoes you habitually wear and consider if they are good for your back. More information on footwear is given on pp. 62–64 and 66. There is so much choice these days that this does not mean that you have to look dowdy! Have good support in the instep – even indoors. Unsupportive, flat slippers prevent your feet working properly, and if your feet start to give you problems, causing you to limp a bit, your back will not like it. If walking is painful for some reason, you can tone up the muscles by *walking* in a swimming pool. The movement will help to straighten your back. Consult a chartered physiotherapist (*see* p. 96) to see if help can be given to ease pain in your legs or feet.

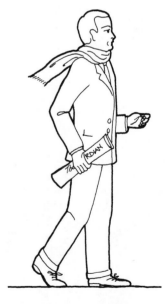

Fig. 6.1 Go for a walk every day – swing your arms to loosen your back.

Seating

If your back is uncomfortable when you sit and/or when you get up from a chair, you may be able to help this by having some support in your low back to prevent it from bending. Sitting in soft, low chairs encourages a stooped posture, so try to interrupt periods of sitting by getting up and walking a little – change the television channels on the set itself rather than by remote control! To prevent your low back seizing up when you are sitting, try doing a few 'pelvic tilts' (*see* Fig. 2.17 on p. 16) every hour or so.

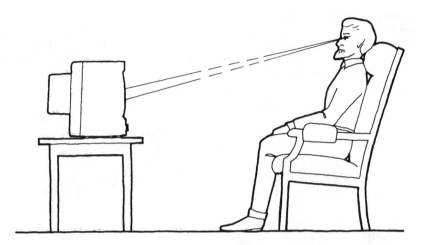

Fig. 6.2 Make sure you are directly facing the screen, not twisted to one side.

Figure 6.2 shows a suitable chair for watching television. A good chair, like this, is easy to get out of because it is not too low. The upholstery is firm without being too hard and there is support for the neck and low back. Note that the television is on a table, not on the floor, so it is not necessary to bend forwards in order to see the screen. If your chair is too low for you, chair-raising blocks are available (address of supplier on p. 96).

Lifting and pushing

Be sensible about your lifting capacity (Fig. 6.3) and protect your back by tightening your tummy muscles before you lift (*see* Fig. 1.17 on p. 7) or push (Fig. 6.4). Back injuries in older people tend to take longer to clear up so it is better to be safe than sorry.

Looking after grandchildren

From a very early age, insist that they climb up on to a chair before you lift them. They soon learn! Avoid carrying them any distance: it isn't worth the risk. Carrying has the same effect on your back as lifting. Older backs cannot cope with sudden jerks, and children do have a habit of jerking.

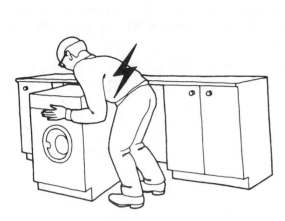

Fig. 6.3 Get help to move heavy objects.

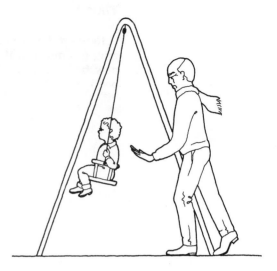

Fig. 6.4 Remember to tighten your tummy muscles.

Gardening

Bending, lifting/carrying and over-reaching are the three things that can trigger off back complaints in gardeners, so sometimes you need to reconsider the layout of your garden and existing types of plants to prevent you over-straining, without spoiling the enjoyment of having a garden. More shrubs and herbaceous perennials instead of annual bedding plants help to avoid too much bending and watering, and ground-cover saves having to weed. Keep the beds narrow to avoid having to lean over to water them. Raised flower beds can be very attractive filled with plants like geraniums that do not need constant watering, but they are expensive to build. Change jobs in the garden frequently to give your back a rest.

Lightweight and long-handled garden tools which give extra leverage are often available at local garden centres (addresses of suppliers are also listed in *Gardening with Arthritis: A Booklet for Patients* – *see* References on p. 96). Many people, young and not so young, find a kneeler helpful in the garden.

If mowing the lawn presents problems, a lifter's belt, worn over clothing, may help (Fig. 6.5). When your back feels sensitive, don't use the grass box. Having the area paved is another option: you can leave spaces between some of the slabs for plants.

A hose-pipe ban when the summer is dry often causes problems when you have to carry lots of water in watering-cans and buckets. One way of making maximum use of available water is to sink a flower-pot to the rim in the earth next to a plant and fill the pot with water so that the roots are watered without wastage. Covering the earth, once watered, with shredded bark reduces evaporation. It is worth consulting your local garden centre regarding which plants come to no harm if they dry out for a few days. Moisture-retentive crystals are also available to reduce the amount of watering required.

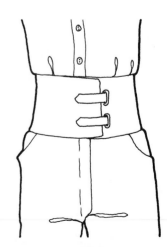

Fig. 6.5 Use a lifter's belt for extra support.

Your bed

A too-hard bed can be uncomfortable, but check that your bed isn't sagging too much. If it is, you may just need a new mattress rather than a new bed. (Also *see* Figs 3.13–3.15 for the best way to get in and out of bed.)

7

Your questions answered

Q. Is my pain muscular?
A. No matter which structure is causing you to have back pain, the muscles themselves will react to it. They go into spasm to protect the spine. With early back and neck problems, *aching* may indeed be caused by overworked muscles. However, with more long-standing problems, the muscles alone are less likely to be the only culprit.

Q. Should I take tablets for the pain?
A. If you are in acute pain which is aggravated by the slightest movement, and cannot find a comfortable position, or if your sleep is disturbed by the pain, your doctor will prescribe appropriate tablets for this. But don't rely on pain-killers to numb the pain while you do the wrong things to your back! Anti-inflammatory tablets are often useful with some chronic arthritic conditions, although some of them have unpleasant side-effects. Your doctor may suggest muscle relaxants, which can stop the nasty twinges of pain caused by the muscles being in spasm.

Q. What will an X-ray show?
A. An X-ray shows up *bone*, not soft tissues such as muscles, ligaments, nerves and discs. Most people from middle-age onwards have some 'wear and tear' in their joints which will show up on an X-ray. If the 'wear and tear' is severe, usually the vertebral bodies will be closer together showing that the disc has narrowed, but again this is part of the normal ageing process.

The radiation dose of a back X-ray is quite high, which is why doctors are reluctant to ask for one routinely.

Q. What is a scan?
A. A scan is a non-invasive procedure which gives more useful information than an X-ray on the state of the spine. There are two types: a CT scan (computerized tomography) and MRI (magnetic resonance imaging). Of the two, the MRI is the more useful. It can show if there are problems with the discs, facet joints and nerves. It is not routinely carried out because it is very expensive.

Q. Is sexual intercourse dangerous when you have a bad back?
A. As the saying goes, 'Where there's a will, there's a way'! Obviously when your back is acutely painful, any energetic exercise is not recommended. Once the pain has settled down, however, try and choose a position that does not provoke your back pain. For instance, if arching your back makes the pain worse, you may be better underneath your partner

(maybe with a pillow under your buttocks) or lying on your side; if bending is more painful you will probably be better on top.

Q. What is osteoporosis?
A. Osteoporosis is a reduction in bone salts, causing 'brittle bones'. It is more common in women than men and is associated with a hormone deficiency after the menopause. This is why doctors often recommend hormone replacement therapy (HRT). If osteoporosis is quite marked, it does show up on an X-ray. You are less likely to get osteoporosis if you take regular exercise and eat healthily.

Q. Does tension cause backache?
A. Most conditions are made worse by tension, and backache is no exception. Tension alone does not *cause* backache, but it increases the resting tone of the muscles, especially in the neck. This then compresses the joints, leading to pain. People are drawn to different ways to relieve tension, such as meditation (which has now been scientifically proven to be an antidote to stress), relaxation classes, listening to music, having counselling, reading, exercising etc. Try to make room in your day for one of these. I teach some of my patients the following relaxation exercise; it only takes a few minutes to do and it is surprising the difference it makes.

Relaxation exercise

This can be done in any position that is comfortable for you but it is probably better done sitting in a chair with your back well supported and with your hands in your lap. Let your shoulders sink down and relax. Now gently place one hand on the front of your waist, and be aware of your breathing. As you breathe in, allow the air to fill your chest so that you expand, like a balloon, round your waist (*see* Fig. 4.1). You should feel your hand gently being pushed outwards. Breathe in to a count of four. Now slowly and effortlessly breathe out to a count of six: you should now feel your hand coming in towards your body. Continue breathing like this for a minute.

Now put your hand back in your lap and attend to each of the five senses in turn:

- Start with the sense of touch. Stay still, and just feel where your body touches the chair. Feel your feet on the floor, the air on your face.
- Next be aware of the sense of taste in your mouth.
- Now the sense of smell.
- Now be aware of the sounds around you. Let the sounds come to you. Listen to the furthest sound.
- Finally just be aware of forms and colours.

Now turn your attention back to relaxed, deep breathing. You may find it easier to close your eyes when experiencing the first four senses.

Try to practice this exercise twice a day, and whenever you are feeling stressed.

Q. Why should I get backache if my back movements are good?
A. The low back tends to be a 'dumping ground' for problems in the legs and feet. For example, if you have flat feet, this can give you backache, which doesn't always come on when you are standing (*see* p. 63).

Occasionally internal organs such as the womb or prostate can 'refer' pain to the back; your doctor or a chartered physiotherapist would be able to reassure you about this.

Q. Would physiotherapy help?
A. Physiotherapy in the form of gentle manipulation, electrical treatment, exercise ('back school'), hydrotherapy or traction often helps people to get over a bout of back or neck pain. Some physiotherapists also use acupuncture, which can be very effective for pain relief. If you are in any doubt about your condition, go to see a *chartered* physiotherapist, i.e. one who is properly qualified (*see* address on p. 96).

Q. Back pain runs in my family. How can I prevent my children getting it?
A. Mainly by setting a good example. Children tend to copy their parents' posture. Make sure you have good seating in the home, which is the right size for *them*. A good chair for young children is the Trip Trapp: it is adjustable, so that it 'grows' with the child. Swimming is the best exercise for children, and activities like T'ai Chi which improve balance and co-ordination as well as strength and flexibility are also good.

Q. Does cold weather make backache worse?
A. Yes, it certainly can, because our muscles automatically tense up. Also, we have primitive receptors in our joints which register changes in atmospheric pressure, so it's not an old wives' tale that some people can feel it in their back when the weather is going to change. It is important to wrap up well in cold weather – make sure you wear a vest, and a scarf to keep your muscles warm. When there is a drop in temperature at night, the tendency is for us to curl up into a ball to keep warm. Your back may not like the after-effect of this, so be prepared for colder weather.

Q. How can I prevent a recurrence of back or neck pain?
A. The first rule of prevention is to get the surfaces that support your body correct. Whatever we are doing, we are mainly standing, walking, sitting or lying down to do it. When standing and walking, our bases of support are our feet, so pay particular attention to your footwear as this can affect your back (*see* p. 62). When sitting for long periods, always sit in a supportive chair (*see* pp. 56–61) rather than a saggy settee. When lying down, choose a bed that supports your back (*see* pp. 49–51).

Maintenance exercises

Keep up two of the exercises that helped you most during your recovery from back pain, and do them every day. Remember that your spine is supported from the front by your abdominal muscles: when you master the abdominal bracing exercise shown in Fig. 1.17, it can be done when you are sitting, standing or walking – it provides a 'muscular corset' to protect your back. These exercises should be carried out only if they do not produce pain. With time, our backs change and sometimes it is necessary to have exercises checked by a chartered physiotherapist to make sure that they are still the right ones.

You may have more questions, but the book ends here. Maybe just reading this book has made you question more. Just remember that although there are people 'out there' who may know the answers, it is *your* body. *Listen* to it and be guided by it. Good luck in your endeavours to keep your Back In Line.

References

Gardening with Arthritis: A Booklet for Patients. Obtainable from The Arthritis and Rheumatism Council, Copeman House, St Mary's Court, St Mary's Gate, Chesterfield, Derbyshire S41 7TD. Tel. 01246-558033.

Joint Hypermobility: A Booklet for Patients. The Arthritis and Rheumatism Council (address as above).

McKenzie, R.A. (1981). *The Lumbar Spine: Mechanical Diagnosis and Therapy.* Spinal Publications, Halifax.

Nachemson, A. (1976). The lumbar spine: an orthopaedic challenge. *Spine,* **1**, 59–71.

Useful addresses

The Chartered Society of Physiotherapy, 14 Bedford Row, London WC1R
   4ED. Tel: 0171 242 1941, Fax: 0171 306 6611.
The Organisation of Chartered Physiotherapists in Private Practice, 8 Weston
   Chambers, Weston Road, Southend-on-Sea, Essex SS1 1AT. Tel: 01702
   392124, Fax: 01702 392125.

Stockists

The Langer Biomechanics Group (UK) Ltd., Brookhouse Way, The Green,
   Cheadle, Stoke-on-Trent, Staffs ST10 1RL. Tel: 01538 755861, Fax: 01538
   755862 (for names of chartered physiotherapists specializing in
   orthotics).
Posturite (UK) Ltd, PO Box 468, Hailsham, East Sussex BN27 4LZ. Tel:
   01323 833353, Fax: 01323 833999.
Spinal Publications Ltd, Unit 1C, Mill Fold Way Industrial Park,
   Ripponden, Halifax HX6 4HS. Tel: 01422 824910, Fax: 01422 824938.
The Back Store, 330 King Street, Hammersmith, London W6 ORR. Tel:
   0181 741 5022, Fax: 0181 741 0683.

Common Complaints Treated by Chartered Physiotherapists

+ **SPINAL PROBLEMS** – including prolapsed discs, degeneration, sciatica, lumbago, stiff/painful neck and referred arm and leg pains.
+ **JOINT PROBLEMS** – arthritis, injury, pain / swelling / stiffness in joints such as shoulders, elbows, wrists, hips, knees and ankles.
+ **INJURIES** – to muscles, ligament, cartilage and tendon problems. Work related conditions such as Repetitive Strain Injury (RSI).
+ **AFTER SURGERY** – rehabilitation after orthopaedic surgery e.g. hip and knee replacements or general physiotherapy after general surgery.
+ **FRACTURES** – treatment to increase the healing rate and to gain full function once the bones have healed.
+ **ABDOMINAL PROBLEMS** – such as spastic colon, colitis and irritable bowel syndrome.
+ **GYNAECOLOGICAL CONDITIONS** – including stress incontinence, salpingitis and post surgery rehabilitation.
+ **OBSTETRICS** – including ante- and post-natal classes / exercise / relaxation / advice and treatment for backpain during pregnancy.
+ **CHEST CONDITIONS** – both medical and surgical, including hayfever, asthma and sinusitis, pneumonia, cystic fibrosis, emphysema, bronchitis and bronchiectasis.
+ **NEUROLOGICAL CONDITIONS** – such as strokes, head injuries, nerve injuries, multiple sclerosis, shingles, cerebral palsy and ME.
+ **PAEDIATRICS** – for childhood conditions including postural and walking problems.
+ **CIRCULATORY PROBLEMS** – such as Raynaud's disease, wounds, ulcers, cardiac rehabilitation.

Chartered PhysioFirst physiotherapists will treat the problem and, by spending time with the patient, will often be able to show them how to help prevent the problem from happening again.

Why see an independent physiotherapist –

- · specialist expertise
- · convenience
- · flexibility
- · speed of service
- · individual attention and treatment

Early treatment can mean a quicker recovery with less time off work. An independent physiotherapist can often provide treatment within 24 hours.

A physiotherapist takes the wider view of a patient's lifestyle to treat the condition and avoid a recurrence – a truly holistic approach.

Physiotherapy is the orthodox therapy – there are a growing number of complementary forms of medicine and the treatment methods they use differ widely.

Most of the basic theories and principals which govern them are included as standard practice in physiotherapy.

What is PhysioFirst?

PhysioFirst is a name that can only be used by Chartered Physiotherapists who are members of The Organisation of Chartered Physiotherapists in Private Practice (OCPPP). There are over 2800 PhysioFirst Centres throughout the UK.

OCPPP
8 Weston Chambers
Weston Road
Southend-on-Sea
Essex SS1 1AT
01702 392124